30-MINUTE
Paleo

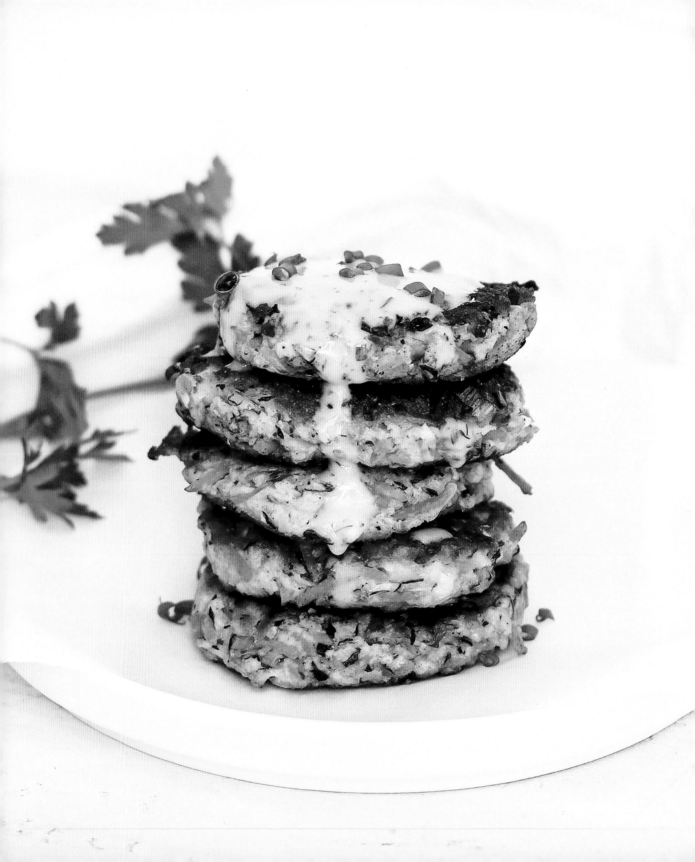

30-MINUTE
Paleo

60 LOW-PREP, BIG-FLAVOR MEALS
FOR EVERY DAY OF THE WEEK

Jessie Bittner

AUTHOR OF *THE SIMPLE PALEO KITCHEN*

PAGE STREET
PUBLISHING CO.

PAGE STREET
PUBLISHING CO.

First published in 2022 by

Page Street Publishing Co.

27 Congress Street, Suite 1511

Salem, MA 01970

www.pagestreetpublishing.com

Distributed by Macmillan, sales in Canada by The Canadian Manda Group.

26 25 24 23 22   1 2 3 4 5

ISBN-13: 978-1-64567-534-1

ISBN-10: 1-64567-534-3

Library of Congress Control Number: 2021937902

Cover and book design by Rosie Stewart for Page Street Publishing Co.

Photography by Jessie Bittner

Printed and bound in the United States of America

THIS BOOK IS DEDICATED TO MY TWO BABY BOYS, HUDSON AND FORD.

Boys: If I could write this book start to finish with the two of you running (and crawling) wild through the house all day, then I have full faith that you can do anything! Know that I love you both so much and will always be your number-one fan, no matter what.

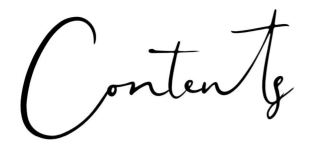

Contents

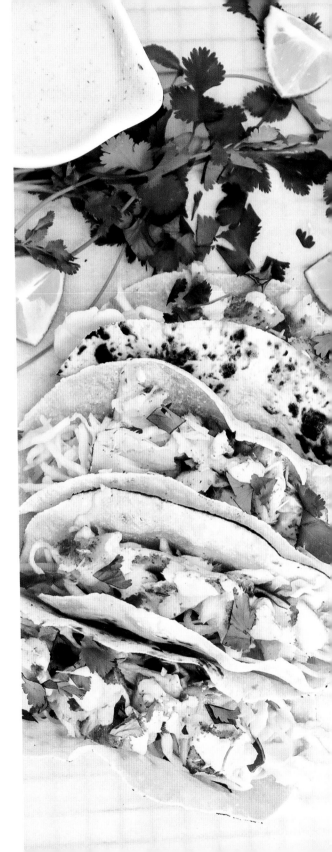

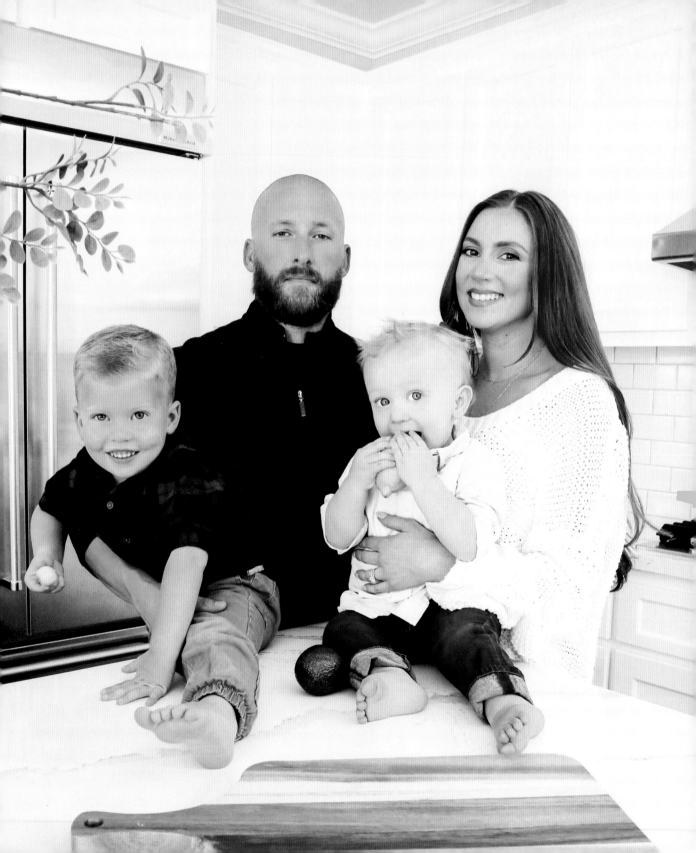

INTRODUCTION

Through all of the years of trial and error, a Paleo-based diet has remained my safe bet for keeping me full and satisfied, but also feeling my very best. Now as a busy working mom of two small boys who are home with me full time, I feel more passionate than ever about getting a healthy meal on the table, yet I have less time than ever. Enter the beauty of a 30-minute (or less) Paleo meal: flavorful, family-friendly dishes that come together in such a short time from start to finish. Get ready for the ultimate guide to delicious food, inspired by my favorite cuisines from all over the world and made with simple, wholesome ingredients.

"Thirty minutes" means from the time you start chopping until the meal is done and plated—and honestly, most of the recipes in this book take even less time than that! I can't tell you how many nights I've checked the time and realized it's 6:00 p.m. and I have nothing planned for dinner. My husband will come back 30 minutes later expecting takeout on the table, and I feel like a superhero with a beautiful, balanced meal ready for all.

When it comes to flavor, I pulled inspiration from all around the globe with these recipes! From Asia to the Mediterranean to the United States' Southwest—even the tropics! I've got you covered with some mouthwatering dishes that will expand your palates in a tasty, crowd-pleasing way. Let's face it— I have to make food that is enjoyable for myself and my husband, but that picky kids will also eat.

While everything in this book is diverse and delicious, the ingredients are also simple. I love achieving new and fun flavors without any difficult-to-source or "only use once" ingredients. It's like a challenge to see what a variety I can create in my kitchen with my same old pantry staples and a few fresh elements. I want my food to be exciting and I want to introduce my family to lots of different flavors, but I don't want the dishes to be complicated (or I honestly won't make them, ha-ha!).

To keep things simple and menu planning–friendly, I divided the chapters by protein. You'll find my favorite quick and easy recipes with easy-to-source poultry, meats and seafood—chicken, ground turkey, steak, salmon and shrimp.

Paleo eating can be sustainable and enjoyable when you've got something delicious to set on the table. Whether it's a comfort food classic, a shortcut for an old favorite or a "takeout fake-out," I hope you'll find a few of our go-to meals to add to your rotation. For my meatless friends, or for those looking for a killer side dish or base for their beloved grilled protein, take a peek at the plant-based recipes (page 77). Some of my hands-down favorites are hiding out there—and you'll be amazed at how satisfying they can be! I've also got brunch covered with both sweet and savory dishes beautiful enough for entertaining, but practical enough for meal prep (page 99). And don't you skip over the soups and salads (page 121)—they are some of my top hearty meals, not starters!

I can't wait for you to get some of our favorite dishes cooking in your kitchens! These recipes are all brand-new for this book, yet have all been on heavy rotation in my home. Even on the busiest nights—when work runs late and we're just home from soccer practice with bath time awaiting and no dinner plans—I take a deep breath and remember I've got a quick, healthy Paleo meal up my sleeve that everyone's gonna love. The best feeling!

I truly hope you enjoy these recipes, from my kitchen and family to yours.

Jessie Bittner

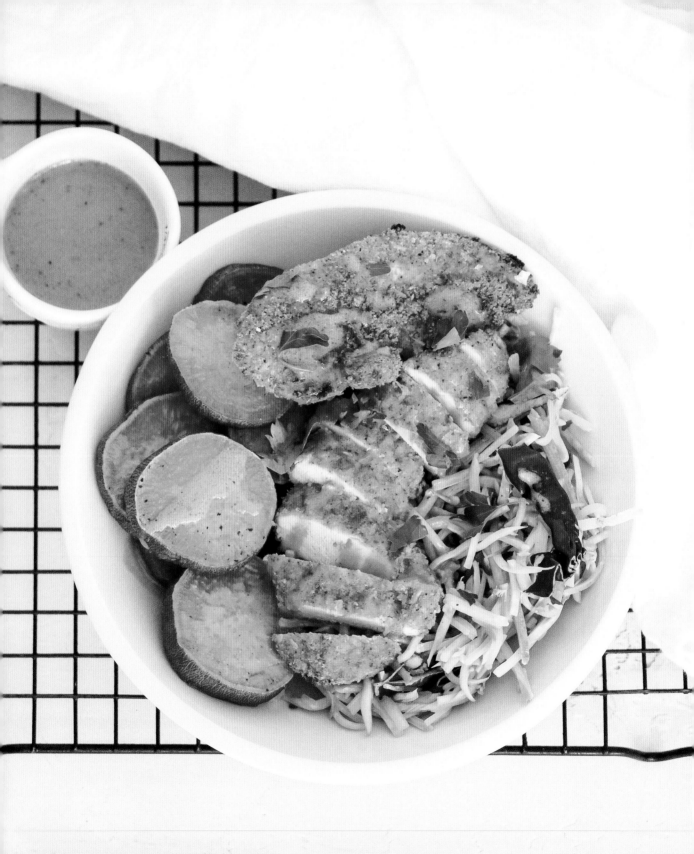

POULTRY ON THE FLY

I love chicken and turkey for easy, accessible meats that everyone can enjoy—but let's be honest . . . they both need some love and flavor to truly be craved! In this chapter, I've got ten delicious ways to whip up some juicy poultry dishes in no time at all. From crispy chicken tenders to one-pan comfort food wonders, I've got you covered!

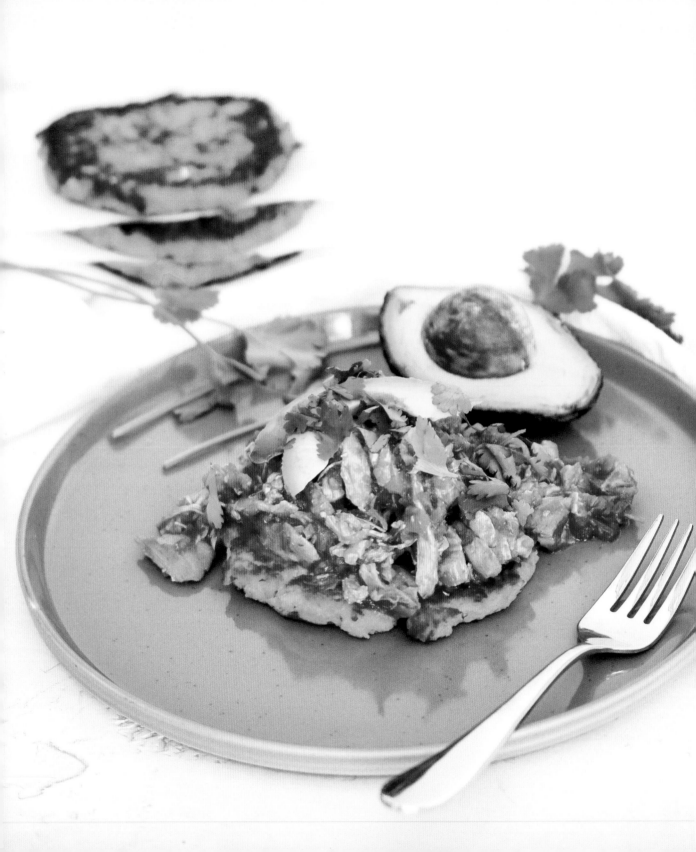

SALSA CHICKEN & SWEET POTATO 'TAMALE' STACKS

Fresh chicken plus a jar of salsa equals a match made in heaven, giving you easy, flavorful chicken that stays super juicy and can be served up in so many ways—and this stovetop version is the quickest. Scooped over my tamale-inspired sweet potato fritters, the combo is the perfect sweet and savory bite with a kick of heat. It has so much flavor, no one will guess you made this in under 30 minutes!

YIELD: 6 STACKS
PREP TIME: 5 MINUTES
COOKING TIME: 18 MINUTES

4 tsp (20 ml) avocado oil, divided

1–1½ lbs (454–681 g) boneless, skinless chicken thighs

2 cups (480 ml) salsa

½ tsp cumin

½ tsp chili powder

Flesh from 2 medium, fully cooked sweet potatoes (about 2 cups [400 g])

1 egg

¼ cup (25 g) almond flour

¼ tsp salt, plus more to taste

¼ tsp black pepper

Chopped cilantro and sliced avocado, for garnish

Heat 2 teaspoons (10 ml) of avocado oil in a heavy-bottomed skillet or Dutch oven over medium-high heat. Add the chicken thighs, and cook for 3 to 4 minutes per side, until they are golden brown and flip easily. Pour the salsa over them and add the cumin and chili powder. Stir to combine, then cover with a lid and cook for 10 minutes, or until the chicken is cooked through.

While the chicken cooks, make the sweet potato tamale fritters. Put the sweet potato flesh in a medium mixing bowl. Use a fork to mash until soft, then add the egg, almond flour, salt and pepper. Mix until combined.

Heat the remaining 2 teaspoons (10 ml) of avocado oil in a skillet over medium heat. Use a ¼-cup (60-ml) measuring cup to scoop out portions of the sweet potato mixture. Using your hands, form a flattened cake about 4 inches (10 cm) wide and ½ inch (1.3 cm) thick. Place in the hot oil and cook for 3 to 4 minutes per side, or until golden brown. Season with a little extra salt, if you like, then set aside on a cooling rack lined with a paper towel.

When the chicken has finished cooking, use two forks to shred it. Serve it scooped over the sweet potato fritters, topped with chopped cilantro and sliced avocado.

QUICK TIP: Keep baked sweet potatoes on hand in the fridge, ready for easy meals like this! If you're not prepped ahead, try the microwave. Rinse the sweet potatoes, then use a fork to poke a few small holes in each one. Wrap each potato in a damp paper towel, then place them all in the microwave. Cook for 3 minutes per side or until soft.

BAKED CRISPY CHICKEN & SWEET POTATO BOWLS WITH HONEY MUSTARD SLAW

The classic "chicken tenders and fries" gets a nutrient-dense upgrade in this easy oven-baked meal. Crispy chicken and tender sweet potato rounds bake in the oven while you whip up a quick broccoli slaw tossed in the most mouthwatering tangy honey mustard dressing. Serve it all up bowl style—the whole family is going to love it!

YIELD: 4 BOWLS
PREP TIME: 7 MINUTES
COOKING TIME: 23 MINUTES

FOR THE CRISPY CHICKEN

1 egg
½ cup (50 g) almond flour
¼ cup (23 g) unsweetened shredded coconut
1 tsp smoked paprika
½ tsp garlic powder
½ tsp salt
¼ tsp black pepper
¼ tsp cayenne pepper
1 lb (454 g) chicken tenders, or breasts cut into strips

FOR THE SWEET POTATOES

2 medium sweet potatoes
Avocado oil spray
¼ tsp salt
¼ tsp black pepper

FOR THE SLAW

2 tbsp (30 ml) Dijon mustard
2 tbsp (30 ml) apple cider vinegar
2 tbsp (30 ml) olive oil
1 tbsp (15 ml) honey
¼ tsp salt
¼ tsp black pepper
4 cups (340 g) broccoli slaw

Set a rack in the upper third of the oven and preheat the oven to 400°F (204°C). Line two baking sheets with parchment paper and set aside.

To make the chicken: In a shallow bowl, whisk the egg. In another shallow bowl, combine the almond flour, shredded coconut, paprika, garlic powder, salt, black pepper and cayenne to make your breading. Dip the chicken tenders into the egg, one at a time, flipping to coat both sides. Transfer to the breading mixture and flip to coat both sides, pressing the chicken down a bit to really grab the breading. Lay the chicken tenders on the first prepared baking sheet in a single layer with a little space in between each.

To make the sweet potatoes: Slice the sweet potatoes into ¼-inch (6-mm) rounds. Arrange on the second baking sheet in a single layer with space between each. Spray with a light coating of avocado oil, and season with the salt and pepper.

Transfer both sheet pans to the oven, with the chicken on the upper rack, and bake for 10 minutes. Remove both sheet pans from the oven, flip the tenders and the sweet potato rounds, then return to the oven for 10 more minutes.

Set the oven to "broil" for the last 2 to 3 minutes to crisp the chicken tenders, watching closely so the parchment doesn't burn.

To make the honey mustard slaw: While the chicken and sweet potatoes cook, in a large bowl, combine the Dijon mustard, apple cider vinegar, olive oil, honey, salt and pepper, whisking until smooth. Set a small amount to the side if you want extra for drizzling on your finished bowls. Add the broccoli slaw to the dressing and toss to combine.

Serve the chicken, sweet potatoes and broccoli slaw in bowls with a drizzle of honey mustard dressing.

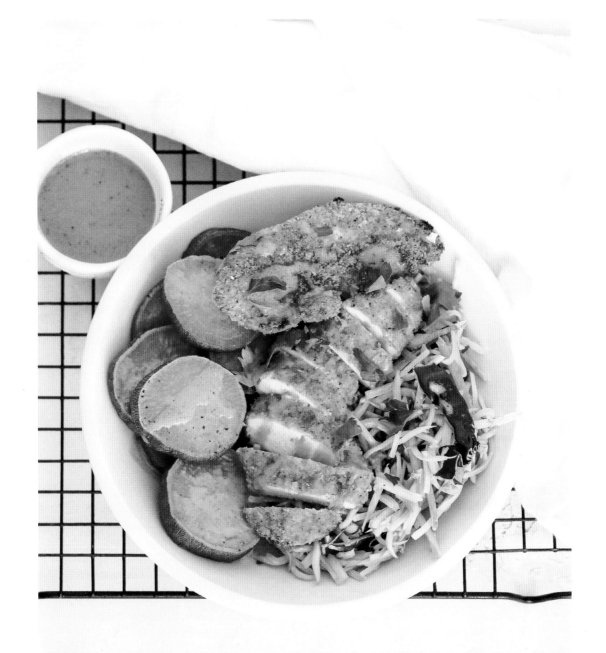

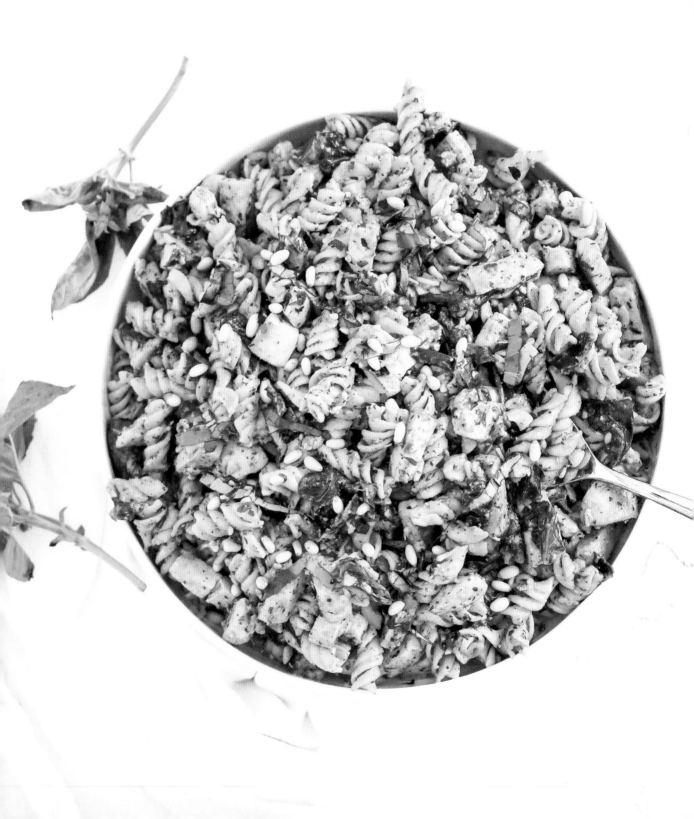

PESTO CHICKEN PASTA WITH SUN-DRIED TOMATOES

There are so many incredible pasta options available now to get a delicious and filling dinner done quick while still keeping it Paleo. From cassava to almond flour to cauliflower, there's bound to be a grain-free version you'll love! Dress it up Italian style with this pantry-friendly dinner that tastes like it's fresh from the garden.

YIELD: 8 CUPS (1.6 KG) OF PASTA
PREP TIME: 5 MINUTES
COOKING TIME: 15 MINUTES

1 lb (454 g) Paleo-friendly pasta (I used rotini)

1 lb (454 g) boneless, skinless chicken breast (about 2 breasts)

1 tbsp (15 ml) olive oil

2 tsp (5 g) minced garlic

½ tsp salt, plus more to taste

½ tsp black pepper

½ tsp dried Italian herb seasoning

¾ cup jarred pesto

¼ cup (14 g) sun-dried tomatoes, julienned

1 cup (23 g) chopped baby spinach

⅓ cup (80 ml) dairy-free milk or cream

¼ cup (34 g) pine nuts, for garnish

¼ cup (10 g) fresh basil, thinly sliced, for garnish

Red pepper flakes, to taste, for garnish (optional)

In a large pot, cook the pasta according to the package instructions until al dente. Drain the pasta, then return it to the pot.

While the pasta cooks, cut the chicken breasts into 1-inch (2.5-cm) pieces. In a large skillet over medium to medium-high heat, heat the olive oil. Add the chicken and minced garlic, then season with the salt, pepper and Italian herb seasoning. Cook for about 7 minutes, until the chicken is lightly browned and cooked through.

When the pasta is finished, add the cooked chicken, pesto, sun-dried tomatoes, baby spinach and milk and stir to combine. Set the heat to medium and cook for 2 to 3 more minutes to warm through.

Serve hot, garnished with pine nuts and sliced fresh basil, plus a pinch of red pepper flakes if you like some heat.

QUICK TIP: Cover the pot of water as you're bringing it to a boil—this helps it heat up faster!

STOVETOP BUFFALO CHICKEN & RICE

There's no better answer to a wild weeknight than a one-dish meal. This skillet version is loaded with creamy Buffalo sauce, tons of sneaky veggies and juicy, golden-brown chicken breast—and it cooks up so quickly. I also love this served chilled, so it's perfect for meal prep or leftovers!

YIELD: 4 SERVINGS
PREP TIME: 5 MINUTES
COOKING TIME: 20 MINUTES

2 tbsp (28 g) ghee, divided

1 lb (454 g) boneless, skinless chicken breast

¼ cup (60 ml) Paleo-friendly mayo

⅓ cup (80 ml) Buffalo sauce

⅓ cup (80 ml) coconut milk

12 oz (340 g) cauliflower rice

2 celery stalks, finely diced

2 large carrots, finely diced

2 cloves garlic, minced

½ tsp salt

½ tsp black pepper

½ tsp garlic powder

½ tsp onion powder

½ tsp smoked paprika

Paleo-friendly ranch dressing and sliced scallions, for garnish

In a large skillet over medium to medium-high heat, melt 1 tablespoon (14 g) of the ghee. Add the chicken breasts and cook for 4 to 5 minutes, or until golden brown. Flip and cook on the other side for an additional 4 to 5 minutes, or until the chicken is cooked through. Transfer the chicken to a plate and set aside.

While the chicken cooks, in a small bowl, combine the mayo, Buffalo sauce and coconut milk and whisk until smooth. Set aside.

When the chicken is done, add the remaining tablespoon (14 g) of ghee to the skillet and heat over medium-high. Add the cauliflower rice, celery, carrots, garlic, salt, pepper, garlic powder, onion powder and paprika. Sauté for 5 to 7 minutes, or until the vegetables are tender-crisp. Return the chicken to the pan and pour the sauce over top. Allow the mixture to simmer over medium heat for 2 to 3 minutes, or until warmed through. Serve hot, garnished with a drizzle of ranch and sliced scallions.

QUICK TIP: I always keep a jar of minced garlic on hand in the refrigerator (and a backup in the pantry!). It's a great way to add flavor without the added time to peel and chop garlic. In addition, I look for the fewest ingredients possible—those usually are the freshest and most flavorful!

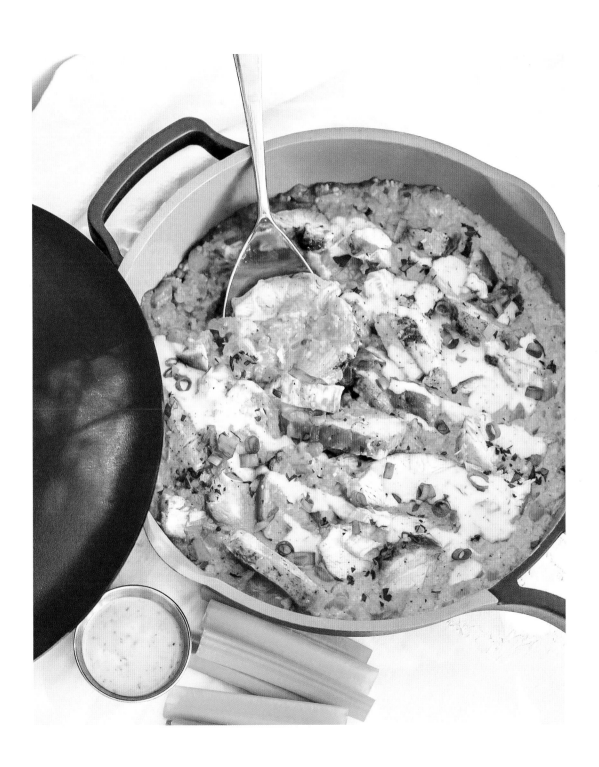

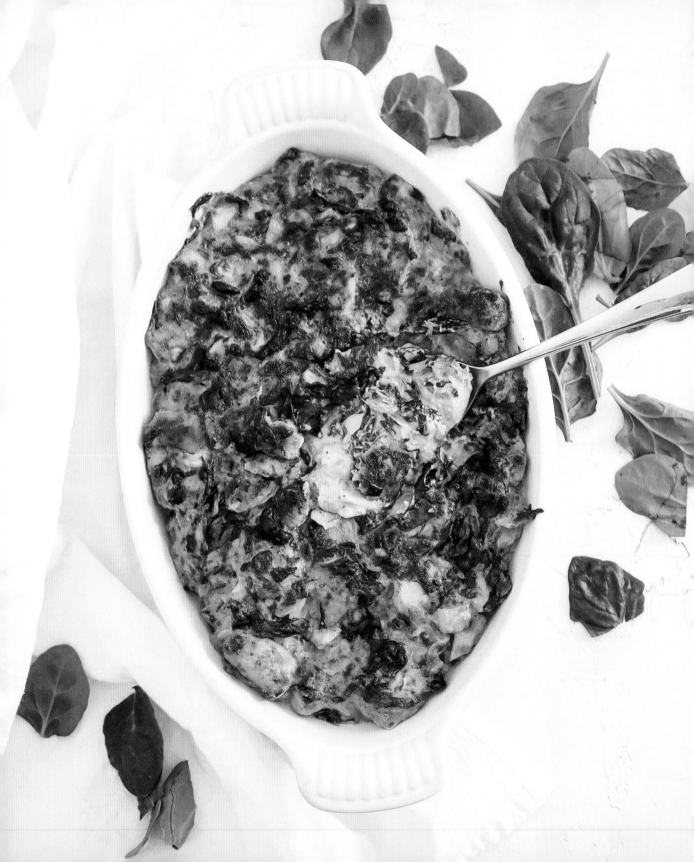

CREAMY SPINACH & ARTICHOKE CHICKEN SKILLET

Warm, bubbly spinach and artichoke dip gets a protein-packed upgrade with this easy skillet. Serve it over greens, use it as a dip for raw veggies or eat it alone by the spoonful. It's crowd-pleasing comfort food at its finest, and one you'll come back to again and again!

YIELD: 4 SERVINGS
PREP TIME: 5 MINUTES
COOKING TIME: 16 MINUTES

1 lb (454 g) boneless, skinless chicken breast

1 tbsp (14 g) ghee

⅔ cup (97 g) raw cashews

½ cup (120 ml) Paleo-friendly mayo

¼ cup (60 ml) chicken broth

½ medium yellow onion, chopped

4 cloves garlic, minced

2 cups (44 g) packed baby spinach

1 (14-oz [400-g]) can artichoke hearts, drained and chopped

½ tsp salt

½ tsp black pepper

Set a rack in the uppermost position in the oven and heat the broiler.

Cut the chicken into 1-inch (2.5-cm) pieces. In a large oven-safe skillet over medium to medium-high heat, melt the ghee. Add the chicken and cook for 8 minutes, or until cooked through, flipping once halfway through. Transfer the cooked chicken to a plate and set aside.

While the chicken cooks, in a high-speed blender or food processor, combine the cashews, mayo and broth. Blend until smooth, 1 to 2 minutes.

When the chicken is done, add the onion, garlic and spinach to the skillet and sauté until the onion is translucent, about 3 minutes. Stir in the artichoke hearts, salt, pepper and cashew cream mixture.

Transfer the skillet to the oven and broil for 3 to 5 minutes, or until golden brown and bubbling.

QUICK TIP: Have a rotisserie chicken on hand? Swap the shredded, cooked chicken for the raw chicken in this recipe and save yourself some extra minutes!

HIBACHI CHICKEN & VEGETABLES WITH YUM-YUM SAUCE

This hibachi-style chicken has all of the restaurant flavor I love, but with no special equipment required. All you need is a large skillet and some high heat, and you're in for a mouthwatering dish—complete with creamy, umami "yum-yum" sauce. This feels special enough for a date night, but is so easy I find myself making it even on the busiest of weeknights!

YIELD: 4 SERVINGS
PREP TIME: 10 MINUTES
COOKING TIME: 15 MINUTES

FOR THE CHICKEN AND VEGETABLES

1 lb (454 g) boneless, skinless chicken breast

1 tbsp (15 ml) toasted sesame oil

4 tbsp (60 ml) coconut aminos, divided

4 cloves garlic, minced

1 tsp minced ginger

1 carrot

1 cup (53 g) cremini mushrooms

1 small yellow onion

1 zucchini

1 tbsp (15 ml) avocado oil

½ tsp salt

½ tsp black pepper

Thinly sliced scallions, for garnish

FOR THE YUM-YUM SAUCE

½ cup (120 ml) Paleo-friendly mayo

1 tbsp (15 ml) coconut aminos

1 tbsp (15 ml) rice vinegar

1 tbsp (16 g) tomato paste

¼ tsp salt

¼ tsp red pepper flakes

¼ tsp garlic powder

¼ tsp onion powder

Cut the chicken breast into bite-sized pieces. In a medium-sized bowl, combine the sesame oil, 3 tablespoons (45 ml) of the coconut aminos, garlic and ginger. Add the chicken pieces and toss to coat. Let it sit for 5 minutes while you cut the vegetables. Thinly slice the carrot. Slice the cremini mushrooms into quarters, then chop up the onion. Finally, halve the zucchini lengthwise before thinly slicing it.

To make the chicken: Heat a large skillet over medium-high heat and pour in the chicken and its sauce. Cook for about 10 minutes, stirring every couple of minutes to brown all sides. Transfer to a plate and set aside.

To make the yum-yum sauce: While the chicken is cooking, make the sauce. In a small bowl, add the mayo, coconut aminos, rice vinegar, tomato paste, salt, red pepper flakes, garlic powder and onion powder and stir until smooth. Set aside for serving.

When the chicken is finished cooking, wipe out the pan and then pour in the avocado oil. Add the carrot, mushrooms, onion, zucchini, remaining 1 tablespoon (15 ml) of coconut aminos, salt and pepper and sauté for about 5 minutes, or until just tender-crisp.

Serve the chicken and vegetables hot with a side of yum-yum sauce for dipping, garnished with sliced scallions.

QUICK TIP: Make a large batch of yum-yum sauce and keep it in the fridge, ready to dress up any quick weeknight stir-fry! It adds so much flavor, and really gives that restaurant-style flair.

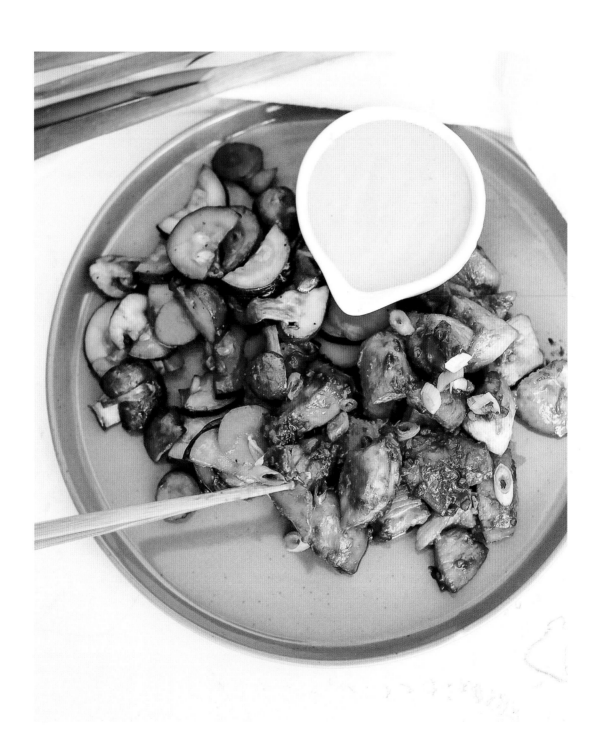

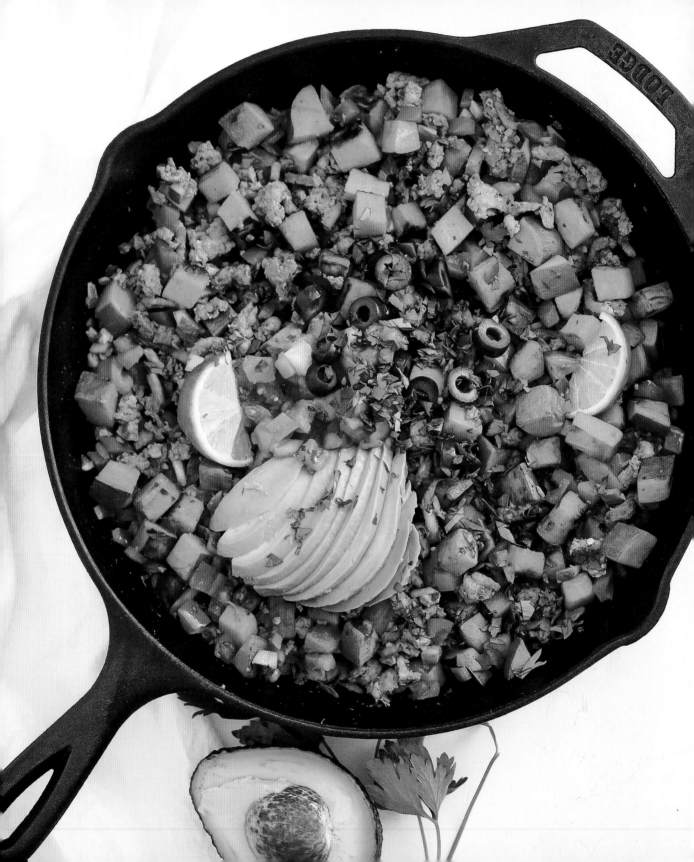

CHIPOTLE TURKEY & SWEET POTATO TACO SKILLET

Ground turkey gets a Tex-Mex makeover in this easy skillet meal. Smoky, spicy chipotle taco flavors are balanced out just right with the hearty sweet potatoes—the combination will make your taste buds sing! Load it up with all of your favorite taco toppings and enjoy this nutrient-dense dish any night of the week.

YIELD: 4 SERVINGS
PREP TIME: 10 MINUTES
COOKING TIME: 11 MINUTES

2 tbsp (30 ml) avocado oil, divided

1 large sweet potato, cut into ½-inch (1.3-cm) cubes (about 3 cups [399 g])

1 lb (454 g) ground turkey

2 tbsp (30 g) taco seasoning

⅛ tsp chipotle powder

1 medium red bell pepper, diced

1 small red onion, diced

2 cloves garlic, minced

1 jalapeño pepper, seeded and minced

¼ cup (4 g) chopped fresh cilantro, for garnish

1 large avocado, sliced, for garnish

½ cup (120 ml) pico de gallo, for garnish

In a large skillet over medium heat, heat 1 tablespoon (15 ml) of avocado oil. Add the cubed sweet potato and cook for 10 minutes, stirring occasionally, until the potato is fork-tender.

While the sweet potato cooks, in a separate large skillet over medium-high heat, pour in the remaining 1 tablespoon (15 ml) of avocado oil. Add the ground turkey, taco seasoning and chipotle powder and cook for 7 to 8 minutes, or until the turkey is crumbled and browned. Add the bell pepper, red onion, garlic and jalapeño and cook for 3 minutes, or until the vegetables are tender.

Stir the sweet potato into the turkey skillet. Serve hot with cilantro, avocado and pico de gallo to garnish.

SHEET PAN MEATBALL DINNER

Meatloaf is a nostalgic childhood favorite of mine—and no one makes it better than mom, right? My mom always used ground turkey, and I love the flavor and light, juicy texture it brings to this classic. Here I make it meatball style to keep things quick and easy, and cook it right alongside a second sheet pan full of broccoli and potatoes. It's a simple comfort food favorite even the kids are going to love!

YIELD: 4 SERVINGS
PREP TIME: 5 MINUTES
COOKING TIME: 20 TO 25 MINUTES

½ cup (120 ml) tomato sauce

2 tbsp (30 ml) balsamic vinegar

1¼ tsp (8 g) salt, divided

¼ tsp red pepper flakes

1 lb (454 g) ground turkey

2 tbsp (30 ml) plus 1 tsp olive oil, divided

¼ cup (25 g) almond flour

½ tsp oregano

½ tsp garlic powder

½ tsp onion powder

1 tsp black pepper, divided

12 oz (340 g) broccoli florets

3 cups (about 440 g) baby gold potatoes, halved

Preheat the oven to 400°F (204°C). Line two baking sheets with parchment paper and set aside.

In a small bowl, combine the tomato sauce, balsamic, ¼ teaspoon of salt and the red pepper flakes and set aside. In a large bowl, combine the turkey, 1 teaspoon of the olive oil, almond flour, oregano, garlic powder, onion powder, ½ teaspoon of salt and ½ teaspoon of pepper with a large fork or your fingers until the ingredients are just mixed. Add half of the tomato sauce mixture to the meat mixture, and stir until combined. Use your hands to roll 20 meatballs, and arrange them in a single layer on one of the lined baking sheets. Top with the remaining half of the tomato sauce mixture.

Arrange the broccoli florets and halved baby gold potatoes on the second baking sheet. Season with ½ teaspoon of salt and ½ teaspoon of pepper and drizzle with the remaining 2 tablespoons (30 ml) of olive oil.

Transfer both dishes to the preheated oven and cook for 20 to 25 minutes, or until the potatoes are fork-tender, the broccoli is crisp and the meatballs are cooked through.

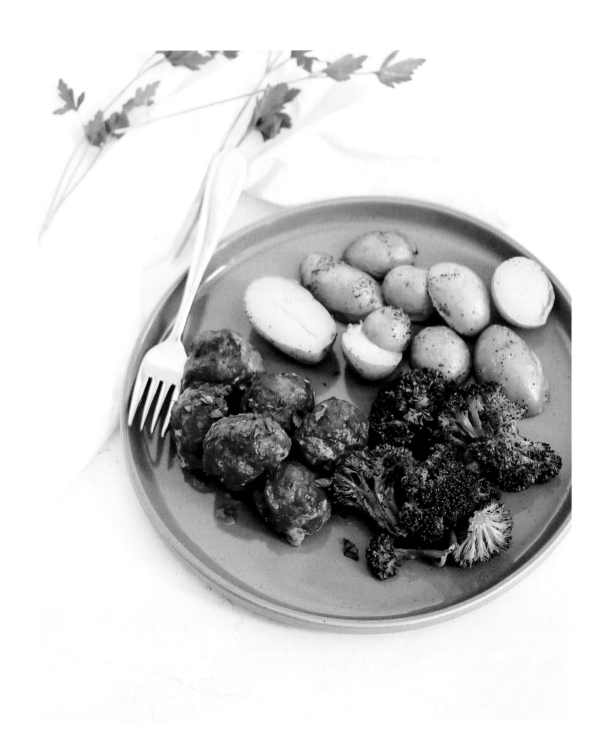

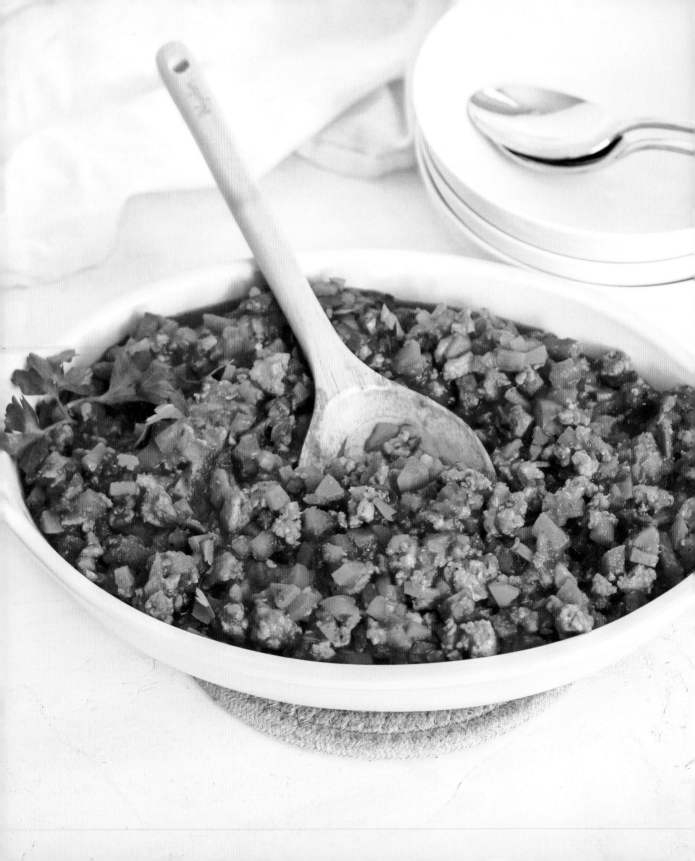

SLOPPY JOE CHILI WITH HIDDEN VEGGIES

Take an extra minute to dice your veggies fine, then watch this savory-sweet skillet come together in no time at all! It's a great way to sneak some extra veggies in and tastes just like a good ol' Sloppy Joe, but loaded with nutrients and free of any refined sugars. Eat it straight from the bowl, or try it served on a gluten-free bun or over a baked potato or sweet potato. The choice is yours!

YIELD: 6 CUPS (1.4 L) CHILI
PREP TIME: 10 MINUTES
COOKING TIME: 15 MINUTES

2 tsp (10 ml) avocado oil

1 lb (454 g) ground turkey

1 red bell pepper, finely diced

1 green bell pepper, finely diced

1 large carrot, finely diced

1 cup (70 g) mushrooms, trimmed and finely diced

½ large yellow onion, finely diced

2 tsp minced garlic

¼ cup (66 g) tomato paste

1 (15-oz [425-g]) can tomato sauce

2 tbsp (30 ml) apple cider vinegar

2 tbsp (30 ml) coconut aminos

1 tbsp (15 ml) coconut sugar or maple syrup

1 tsp onion powder

1 tsp garlic powder

1 tsp chili powder

½ tsp smoked paprika

½ tsp salt, plus more to taste

½ tsp black pepper

In a large skillet over medium-high heat, heat the avocado oil. Add the ground turkey and cook for 5 minutes, or until it's broken into small pieces and just browned. Add the bell peppers, carrot, mushrooms, onion and garlic and sauté for 5 more minutes, or until the vegetables are tender-crisp.

Stir in the tomato paste, tomato sauce, vinegar, coconut aminos, coconut sugar, onion powder, garlic powder, chili powder, smoked paprika, salt and pepper. Reduce the heat to medium-low and simmer for 5 more minutes to combine the flavors and fully soften the veggies. Season with additional salt to taste and serve hot.

MEDITERRANEAN STUFFED TURKEY BURGERS WITH TZATZIKI SAUCE

Loading up turkey burgers with all of the stuffings is a sure way to keep them extra juicy—a trick I learned from my mama! This recipe takes us to the Mediterranean with savory burgers, filled with sun-dried tomatoes and herbs, and a fresh creamy tzatziki sauce to scoop over the top. The sauce also makes a killer salad dressing—so keep that extra on hand in the fridge for lunch the next day!

YIELD: 4 TURKEY BURGERS
PREP TIME: 10 MINUTES
COOKING TIME: 10 TO 12 MINUTES

FOR THE TZATZIKI SAUCE

¼ cup (60 ml) coconut milk

⅓ cup (80 ml) Paleo-friendly mayo

½ medium cucumber, peeled and finely diced

1 tbsp (15 ml) lemon juice

2 tsp (7 g) fresh dill, finely chopped

1 tsp minced garlic

¼ tsp salt

¼ tsp black pepper

FOR THE TURKEY BURGERS

1 lb (454 g) ground turkey

1 cup (30 g) baby spinach, finely chopped

1 tsp minced garlic

1 tsp dried Italian herb seasoning

½ tsp garlic powder

½ tsp salt

½ tsp black pepper

1 large egg

½ cup (27 g) chopped sun-dried tomatoes

⅓ cup (25 g) nutritional yeast

2 tbsp (30 ml) olive oil

Mixed greens, for serving

To make the tzatziki sauce: In a small bowl, combine the coconut milk, mayo, cucumber, lemon juice, dill, garlic, salt and pepper and transfer to the refrigerator.

To make the turkey burgers: In a large bowl, combine the ground turkey, spinach, garlic, Italian herb seasoning, garlic powder, salt, pepper, egg, sun-dried tomatoes and nutritional yeast with a large fork or your fingers until the ingredients are just mixed. Divide the mixture into four round patties about ½ inch (1.3 cm) thick.

In a large skillet over medium to medium-high heat, heat the olive oil. Add the patties, with a little space between each, and cook for 5 to 6 minutes on each side, or until browned and cooked through.

Serve the turkey burgers over a bed of mixed greens and top with the chilled tzatziki sauce.

QUICK TIP: Want to squeeze another quick dinner out of this? Double the burger recipe and store the extra burgers in the freezer to reheat any time!

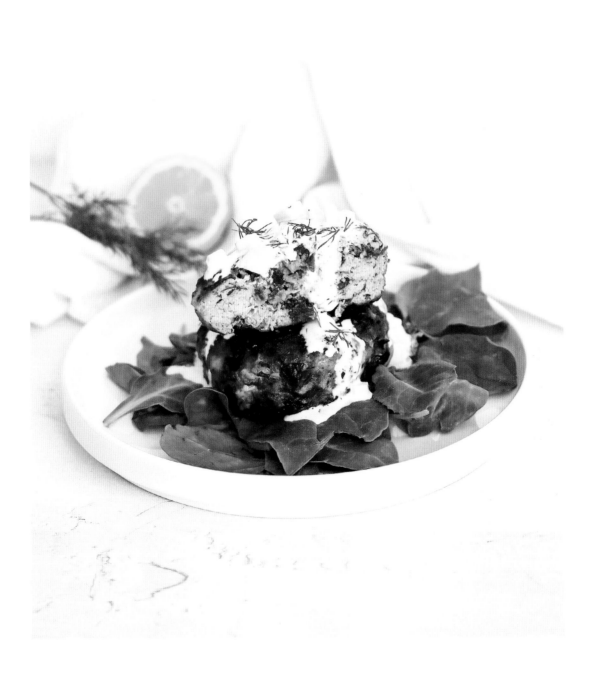

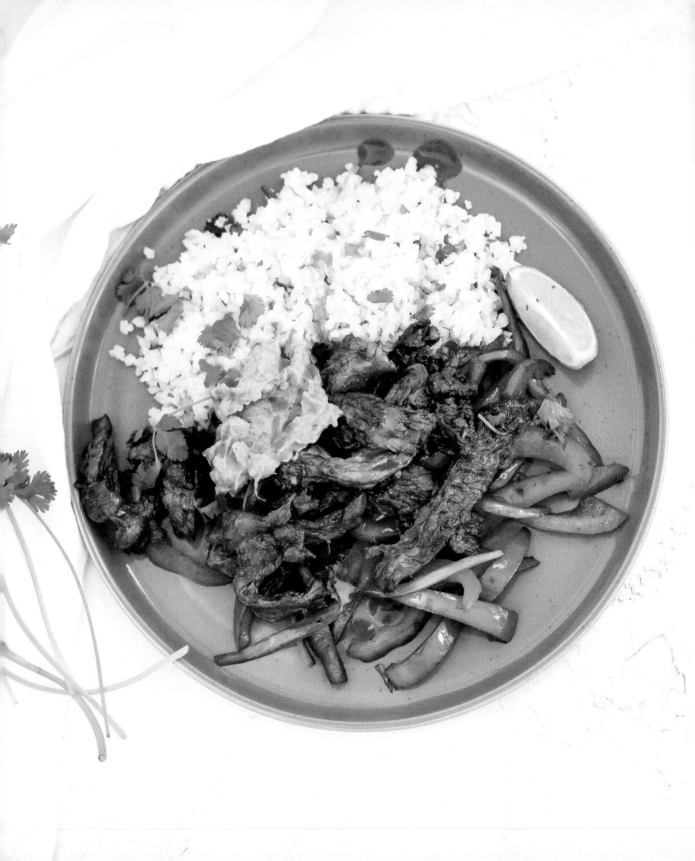

MEATS MADE QUICK

This chapter is full of comfort food favorites featuring beef, pork and sausage with more flavor than anyone would expect to come out of 30 minutes or less. I love hearty, savory dishes for filling up the whole family and making great leftovers—and that's just what these recipes do. From Italian favorites to American classics to a few takeout fake-outs, you're going to love what's up next!

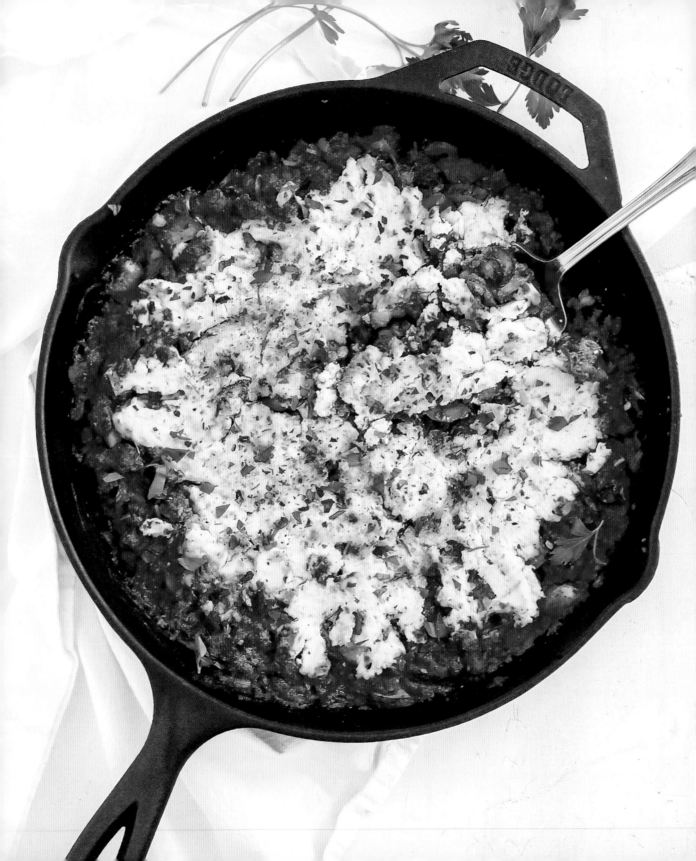

BEEF & VEGETABLE LASAGNA SKILLET

A great lasagna is less about the pasta sheets and more about the rich, meaty tomato sauce, savory veggies and creamy ricotta layers. With this simple skillet, you'll get all of the delicious Italian lasagna flavor and texture you love, but in a fraction of the time!

YIELD: 6 (1-CUP [240-ML]) SERVINGS
PREP TIME: 10 MINUTES
COOKING TIME: 20 MINUTES

2 tsp (10 ml) olive oil

1 lb (454 g) ground beef

½ medium yellow onion, chopped

½ medium red bell pepper, diced

1 medium zucchini, quartered lengthwise then sliced into ¼-inch (6-mm)-thick pieces

1 cup (70 g) trimmed and sliced cremini mushrooms

1 cup (30 g) baby spinach, chopped

1 tbsp (7 g) minced garlic

1 tsp dried Italian herb seasoning

½ tsp salt

½ tsp black pepper

1 (15-oz [425-g]) can tomato sauce

8 oz (225 g) dairy-free ricotta

Finely chopped fresh parsley and red pepper flakes, for garnish

Set a rack in the uppermost position of the oven and preheat the broiler.

In a large ovenproof skillet over medium heat, heat the olive oil. Add the ground beef and cook for 5 to 7 minutes, until browned and crumbled. Adjust the heat to medium-high and add the onion, bell pepper, zucchini, mushrooms, spinach, garlic, Italian herb seasoning, salt and pepper. Sauté, stirring frequently, for 5 minutes, or until the vegetables are tender and the spinach is wilted. Stir in the tomato sauce until combined and continue to cook for 2 to 3 minutes to warm through.

Use a large spoon or rubber spatula to spread the ricotta over top of the skillet in an even layer. Transfer the skillet to the oven and broil for 5 minutes, or until the top is golden brown. Garnish with chopped parsley and red pepper flakes to taste, and serve hot.

QUICK TIP: Want to stretch this into two nights worth of dinner? On night two, prepare a package of Paleo-friendly pasta. Serve the leftover lasagna skillet over top and enjoy!

BUTTERY FLANK STEAK & POTATOES WITH GREEN BEANS

If you're a meat and potatoes lover, you've come to the right place! Start by roasting up your potatoes and green beans all on one baking sheet—they truly cook to tender-crisp perfection in just 20 minutes! Meanwhile, grill up a tender flank steak to your liking. It's an easy cut of meat to work with, and is super tender and delicious when cooked quick and sliced against the grain. Serve it all up with a drizzle of hot herbed butter and devour!

YIELD: 4 SERVINGS
PREP TIME: 5 MINUTES
COOKING TIME: 23 MINUTES

1 lb (454 g) small red potatoes, halved

2 cups (220 g) green beans

3 tbsp (45 ml) avocado oil, divided

Salt

Black pepper

1 lb (454 g) flank steak

1 tsp minced garlic

½ tsp oregano

½ tsp onion powder

¼ cup (56 g) grass-fed butter or ghee

¼ cup (15 g) parsley, finely chopped

Set a rack in the oven and preheat it to 425°F (218°C). Line a baking sheet with parchment paper, then arrange the potatoes on one side and the green beans on the other, all in a single layer. Drizzle with 2 tablespoons (30 ml) of the avocado oil and season with salt and pepper. Transfer to the oven and bake for 20 minutes. Set the oven to broil and cook for an additional 3 minutes to lightly brown the vegetables.

While the vegetables cook, in a grill pan or large cast-iron skillet over medium-high heat, heat the remaining 1 tablespoon (15 ml) of avocado oil. Use a paper towel to pat the flank steak dry, then season both sides with salt and pepper. Add to the hot pan and cook for 3 to 5 minutes on each side, or until the internal temperature of the steak reaches 5 degrees under the final temperature you prefer. Transfer the steak to a cutting board to rest for 5 minutes before slicing against the grain.

In a small saucepan over medium-low heat, heat the butter and parsley until the butter is just melted.

Serve the steak and vegetables hot with a drizzle of the butter over top.

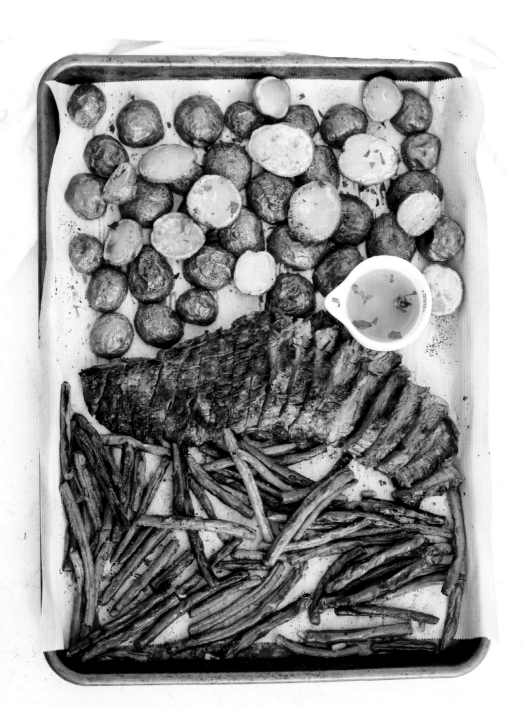

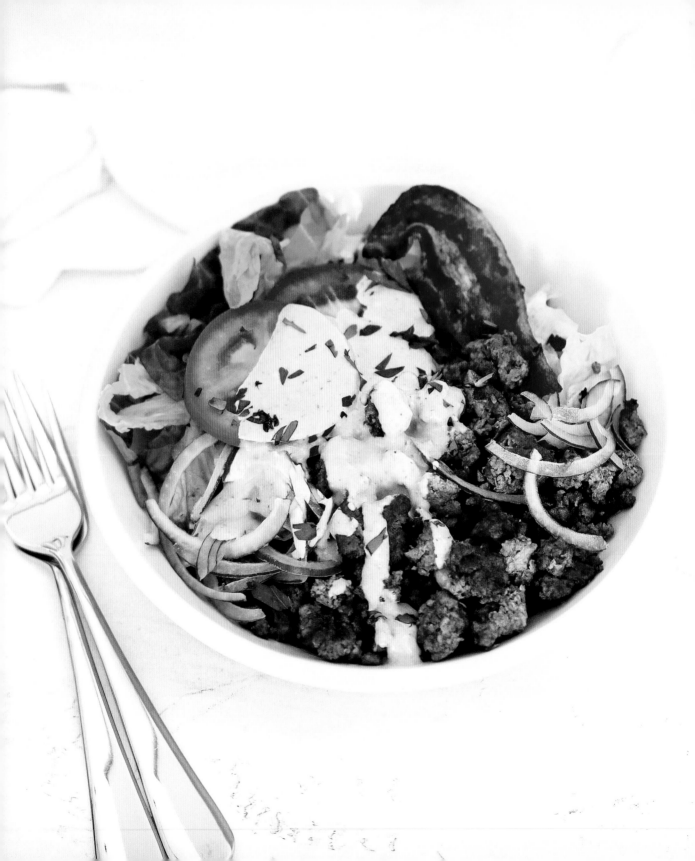

SHORTCUT BURGER BOWLS WITH SPECIAL SAUCE

The easiest way to serve up your favorite burger meat and toppings? Bowl style! Get the perfect ratio of crispy beef, lettuce, bacon, tomato and onion in every bite, and save yourself the mess of a lettuce-wrapped patty. Serve it up in a "build your own bowl" bar so everyone gets exactly what they want on theirs—and don't forget that magical "Special Sauce" to really take these bowls to the next level!

YIELD: 4 BOWLS
PREP TIME: 5 MINUTES
COOKING TIME: 10 MINUTES

2 tsp (10 ml) avocado oil, divided
1 lb (454 g) ground beef
½ tsp salt
½ tsp black pepper

FOR THE SPECIAL SAUCE
½ cup (120 ml) Paleo-friendly mayo
2 tbsp (30 ml) Paleo-friendly ketchup
1 tbsp (15 ml) coconut aminos
2 tsp (4 g) onion powder
½ tsp hot sauce
¼ tsp salt

FOR SERVING
4 cups romaine lettuce, chopped
4 slices cooked bacon
1 large Roma tomato, sliced ¼ inch (6 mm) thick
½ medium red onion, thinly sliced
Finely chopped fresh parsley, for garnish

Heat 1 teaspoon of the avocado oil in a large skillet over medium heat. Add the ground beef, salt and pepper and cook until the ground beef is crumbled and no longer pink, 5 to 7 minutes. Drain any fat, then add the remaining teaspoon of avocado oil. Turn the heat up to high, and brown the beef until it is crispy around the edges, about 3 minutes.

To make the special sauce: While the beef cooks, make the special sauce in a small bowl by combining the mayo, ketchup, coconut aminos, onion powder, hot sauce and salt. Mix until smooth and set aside for serving.

To serve: Divide the romaine lettuce between four bowls. Add the "burger" beef to each bowl, then top with bacon, sliced tomato, sliced red onion and a drizzle of special sauce. Garnish with fresh parsley.

QUICK TIP: We always cook bacon on Sunday mornings and make plenty to keep in the fridge for jazzing up dinners throughout the week. Pop in the microwave or air fryer until crisp, and enjoy!

CARNE ASADA FAJITAS WITH CILANTRO-LIME RICE

Fajitas are a go-to for us. Served bowl style over cauliflower rice or over greens for a fresh salad—it's such a versatile recipe! The trick with this one is cooking the meat right in its marinade. That way, it doesn't matter how long the meat sits ahead of time; just cook that flavor right in! With garlic, chili powder, cumin and lime, your tastes buds will be begging for more of this easy, savory dinner staple.

YIELD: 4 BOWLS
PREP TIME: 10 MINUTES
COOKING TIME: 15 MINUTES

2 tbsp (30 ml) coconut aminos

2 tbsp (30 ml) plus 1 tsp avocado oil, divided

2 tbsp (30 ml) lime juice

2 tsp (17 g) minced garlic

1 tsp chili powder

1 tsp cumin

1 tsp dried oregano

1½ lb (681 g) steak, cut into thin strips (rib eye, skirt steak or flank steak work well)

½ medium red onion, sliced

1 red bell pepper, sliced

1 green bell pepper, sliced

12 oz (340 g) fresh or frozen cauliflower rice

2 tbsp (1 g) chopped cilantro

Juice of ½ lime

½ tsp salt

Guacamole and chopped cilantro, for garnish

In a large bowl, combine the coconut aminos, 2 tablespoons (30 ml) of the avocado oil, lime juice, minced garlic, chili powder, cumin and oregano and whisk together. Add the steak to the bowl as you slice it, and let it marinate at room temperature for at least 5 minutes.

Heat a large skillet over medium-high heat. Add the steak and its marinade to the skillet and cook for 2 to 3 minutes per side, until browned. Transfer the cooked meat to a bowl and set aside.

Add the sliced onion and bell peppers to the same skillet and cook for 4 to 5 minutes, tossing as they cook, until just tender-crisp.

In a medium saucepan over medium-high to high heat, heat the remaining 1 teaspoon of avocado oil. Add the cauliflower rice and cook for 3 to 4 minutes, or until just tender. Turn off the heat and stir in the chopped cilantro, lime juice and salt until just combined.

Serve the fajitas over the cilantro-lime rice, topped with guacamole and chopped cilantro to garnish.

QUICK TIP: Rib eye steaks are one of my favorite cuts to use for quick recipes like this. They thaw super fast, which makes them an easy one to grab from the freezer and defrost night-of. Speaking of frozen foods, we always use frozen cauliflower rice! There's no need to thaw it first, and it has great neutral flavor.

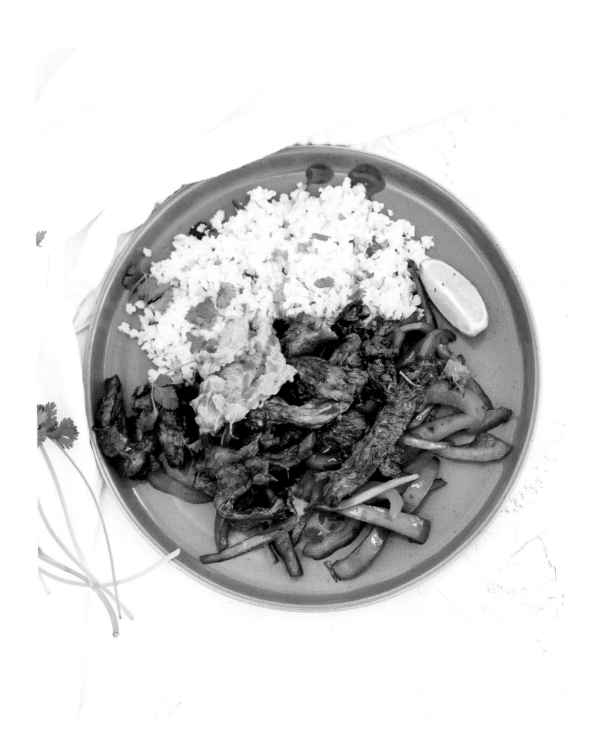

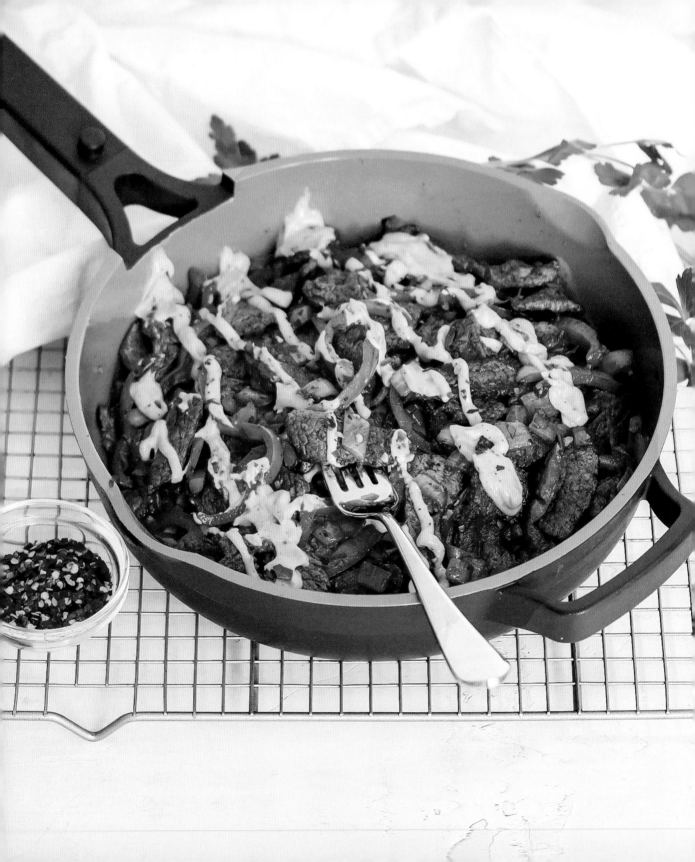

PHILLY CHEESESTEAK SKILLET WITH PALEO CHEESE SAUCE

If you're a family of many food preferences, get ready to please them all with this Philly Cheesesteak Skillet. The crispy thin-sliced beef with tender onions and peppers is so delicious on its own, "protein style," but can easily be served in a toasty roll if your family wants a little extra!

YIELD: 4 SERVINGS
PREP TIME: 10 MINUTES
COOKING TIME: 11 MINUTES

2 tbsp (30 g) ghee, divided

1 large green bell pepper, sliced thin

1 medium sweet onion, large dice

1 tsp minced garlic

1 lb (454 g) sirloin steak, sliced thin

¾ tsp salt, divided

¾ tsp black pepper, divided

½ cup (120 ml) Paleo-friendly mayo

2 tsp (3 g) nutritional yeast

1 tsp coconut aminos

½ tsp garlic powder

In a large skillet over medium to medium-high heat, heat 1 tablespoon (15 g) of the ghee. Add the bell pepper, onion and garlic and sauté for 4 to 5 minutes, or until the vegetables are tender. Transfer the cooked vegetables to a bowl and set aside.

Heat the remaining 1 tablespoon (15 g) of ghee in the skillet and add the thinly sliced steak. Season with ½ teaspoon each of salt and pepper, and cook for about 2 minutes per side, or until just browned. Stir the vegetables back in to warm for an additional 2 minutes.

While the vegetables warm, make your cheese sauce in a small bowl by combining the mayo, nutritional yeast, coconut aminos, garlic powder and the remaining ¼ teaspoon each of salt and pepper. Stir until smooth.

Serve the skillet hot with cheese sauce drizzled over the top.

QUICK TIP: Working with partially frozen steak is actually a blessing in disguise with this recipe, as the steak is a lot easier to slice thin when it's still slightly solid. Use a sharp knife, and cut it as thin as you can! This gets it extra crispy and lets it cook up so quickly.

L'ULTIMO ITALIAN MEATBALLS

Savory, meaty and cooked to tender perfection in your favorite marinara . . . it doesn't get better than these meatballs! You know they're the ultimate when there's no pasta necessary (although you could totally make some and serve it up classic style!). These meatballs are so delicious and filling, we eat them on their own for a whole meal. Pair them with a simple side salad if you like, or simply enjoy!

YIELD: 6 SERVINGS (4 MEATBALLS EACH)
PREP TIME: 10 MINUTES
COOKING TIME: 18 MINUTES

1 lb (454 g) ground beef

1 egg

⅓ cup (32 g) almond flour

2 tbsp (30 ml) chicken broth

¼ cup yellow onion, minced

2 tsp minced garlic

¼ cup (15 g) fresh parsley, finely chopped

1 tsp dried Italian herb seasoning

1 tsp salt

½ tsp black pepper

2 tbsp (30 ml) olive oil

1 (32-oz [900-g]) jar marinara sauce

Chopped fresh parsley and red pepper flakes, for garnish

In a large mixing bowl, combine the ground beef, egg, almond flour, chicken broth, onion, garlic, parsley, Italian herb seasoning, salt and pepper. Use a large fork or your hands to mix until the ingredients are well combined. Using a cookie dough scoop, scoop roughly 3 tablespoons (45 g) of the meatball mixture into your hands. Form the mixture into about 24 meatballs and set aside on a cutting board.

Heat the olive oil in a large skillet over medium-high heat. Add the meatballs to the skillet and cook until browned on all sides, 1 to 2 minutes per side. Pour the marinara sauce over top, and allow the sauce to come to a simmer. Cover the skillet with a lid and cook for 10 minutes, or until the meatballs are cooked through.

Serve hot, garnished with chopped parsley and red pepper flakes.

QUICK TIP: Jarred marinara is a staple in our pantry for throwing together delicious (and fast) weeknight meals. I look for the simplest ingredients possible—always sugar and soy free, and organic if I can. Don't be afraid to jazz it up with a little more garlic powder, red pepper flakes or fresh herbs to really make it your own.

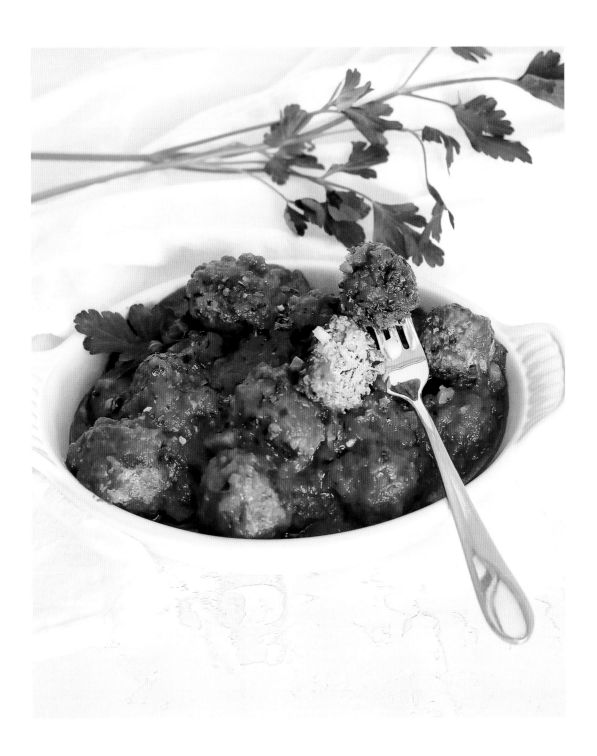

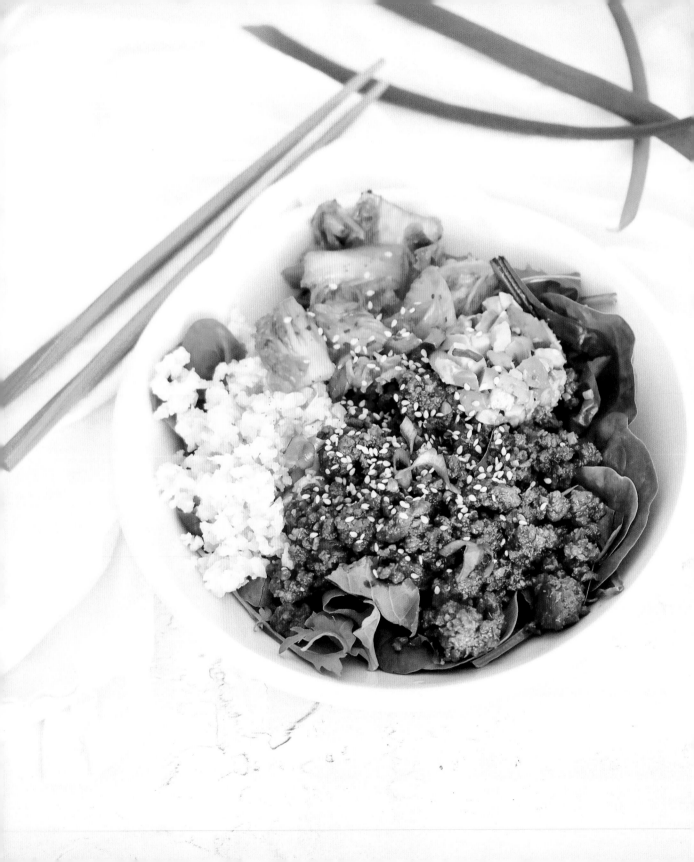

TAKEOUT-STYLE KOREAN BEEF BOWLS

This recipe is inspired by a Korean-Japanese fusion restaurant we used to order from that made the best "rice bowls" loaded up with Korean barbecue beef, spicy kimchi, fresh avocado and crunchy spring mix to balance it all out. Now I love ordering out for a "night off" from the kitchen, but when you can make something this good in under 20 minutes? You'll beat the delivery guy every time!

YIELD: 4 BOWLS
PREP TIME: 3 MINUTES
COOKING TIME: 13 MINUTES

1 tbsp (15 ml) toasted sesame oil

1 lb (454 g) ground beef

1 tsp minced ginger

1 tsp minced garlic

¼ tsp red pepper flakes

2 tbsp (30 ml) rice wine vinegar

3 tbsp (45 ml) coconut aminos, plus more for garnish

1 tbsp (16 g) tomato paste

12 oz (340 g) cauliflower rice

2 cups spring mix

1 cup (150 g) kimchi

1 large avocado, finely chopped

Toasted sesame seeds and thinly sliced scallions, for garnish

In a skillet over medium to medium-high heat, heat the sesame oil. Add the ground beef and cook until crumbled and browned, 5 to 7 minutes. Stir in the ginger, garlic, red pepper flakes, rice wine vinegar, coconut aminos and tomato paste and continue to cook for 3 minutes.

While the beef cooks, put the cauliflower rice in a medium saucepan over high heat. Cook for 3 minutes, or until just tender.

To serve, divide the spring mix among four bowls. Top with the cauliflower rice and beef mixture. Add ¼ cup (38 g) of kimchi and one-fourth of the avocado to each bowl. Garnish with toasted sesame seeds, sliced scallions and an extra drizzle of coconut aminos, if you like.

QUICK TIP: Store-bought kimchi is a great way to add probiotic foods to your diet—and it's delicious! Look for sugar-free options (the spicy kind is my favorite!). Add to any Asian-inspired dishes for extra flavor, texture and health benefits.

SMOTHERED PORK CHOPS WITH SAUTÉED GREENS

Ready for some southern classic comfort food? These pan-fried pork chops are smothered in the most delicious onion gravy that you'll never guess is dairy- and gluten-free. It is rich, indulgent and done in under 25 minutes. Serve with some garlicky sautéed greens and try not to lick the plate clean!

YIELD: 4 SERVINGS
PREP TIME: 5 MINUTES
COOKING TIME: 19 MINUTES

4 thick-cut pork chops

1½ tsp salt, divided

1½ tsp black pepper, divided

3 tbsp (45 ml) avocado oil, divided

½ medium yellow onion, thinly sliced

4 tsp (8 g) minced garlic, divided

½ cup (73 g) raw cashews

2 cups (480 ml) chicken broth

1 tbsp (5 g) nutritional yeast

1 tbsp (15 ml) coconut aminos

¼ tsp cayenne pepper (optional, omit if you don't like heat)

¼ tsp dried thyme

4 cups mixed greens (I use a blend of spinach, chard and kale)

Finely chopped fresh parsley and red pepper flakes, for garnish

Pat the pork chops dry and season both sides with 1 teaspoon each of salt and pepper. In a large skillet over medium-high heat, heat 2 tablespoons (30 ml) of the avocado oil. Add the pork chops and cook for 4 minutes per side, or until golden brown. Transfer to a plate and set aside.

Reduce the heat to medium and add the onion and 2 teaspoons (4 g) of the garlic to the pan. Cook, stirring occasionally, for about 5 minutes, or until soft and golden brown.

While the onions and garlic are cooking, add the cashews, broth, nutritional yeast, coconut aminos, remaining ½ teaspoon each of salt and pepper, cayenne (if using) and thyme to a high-speed blender and pulse until smooth.

Add the pork chops back to the skillet with the onions and garlic, along with any juices from the plate, and pour the sauce over top. Simmer for about 10 minutes, or until the pork chops are cooked through and sauce is warm and bubbling.

While the smothered pork chops cook, heat the remaining 1 tablespoon (15 ml) of avocado oil in a large skillet over medium-low heat. Add the mixed greens and remaining 2 teaspoons (4 g) of garlic and sauté for 5 minutes, or until the greens are just wilted and the garlic is softened.

Serve the smothered pork chops with a side of sautéed greens, with chopped parsley and red pepper flakes to garnish.

QUICK TIP: My favorite sauce is a blender sauce. To make cleaning that blender just as quick and easy, add hot water and a little dish soap to your blender, then blend on high for a minute. Rinse and dry. It will be squeaky clean and ready for the next day's work!

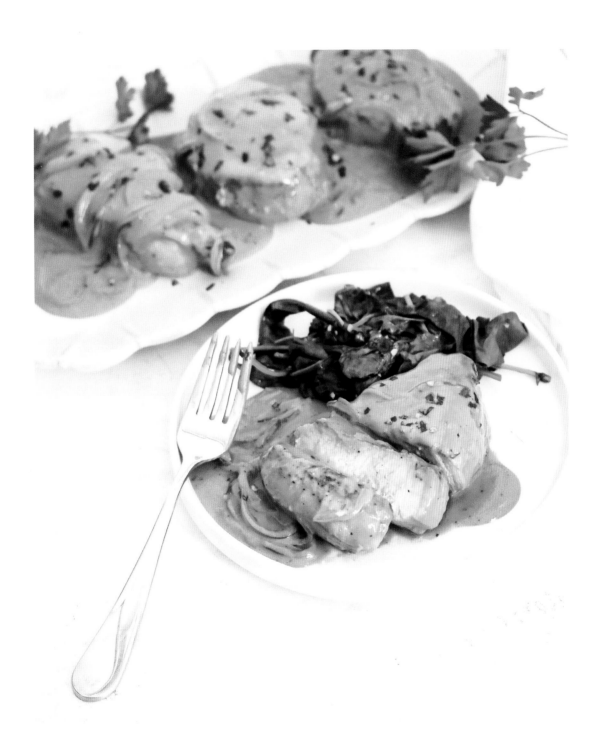

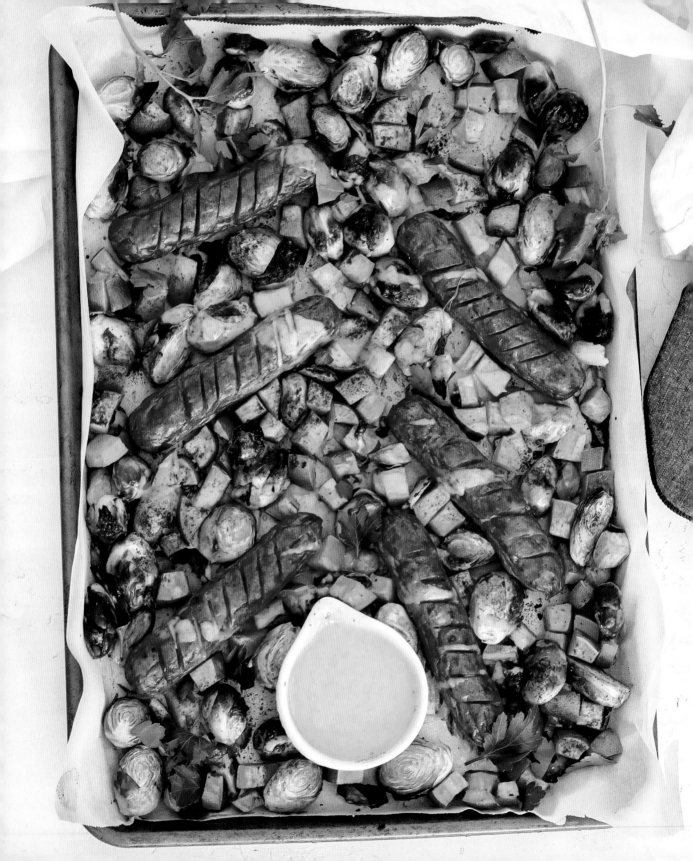

SAUSAGE, SWEET POTATO & BRUSSELS SHEET PAN WITH BUFFALO RANCH

The truest of "one dish" meals, this sausage and vegetable dinner comes together on a single sheet pan with a zesty Buffalo ranch to top it off. Go for any fully cooked sausage you love! Chicken apple can give a sweet-savory vibe, or try something with a little spice to it to kick things up a notch.

YIELD: 4 SERVINGS
PREP TIME: 5 MINUTES
COOKING TIME: 20 MINUTES

2 medium sweet potatoes, cut into ½-inch (1.3-cm) cubes

1 lb (454 g) Brussels sprouts, halved

½ tsp chili powder

½ tsp garlic powder

½ tsp onion powder

½ tsp salt

½ tsp black pepper

1 tbsp (15 ml) avocado oil

12 oz (340 g) fully cooked, Paleo-friendly chicken sausage

3 tbsp (45 ml) Buffalo sauce

3 tbsp (45 ml) Paleo-friendly ranch dressing, plus more for drizzling

Chopped fresh parsley, for garnish

Preheat the oven to 425°F (218°C). Line a baking sheet with parchment paper and arrange the cubed sweet potatoes and halved Brussels sprouts in a single layer. Season with the chili powder, garlic powder, onion powder, salt and pepper and drizzle with avocado oil. Nestle the chicken sausages in among the vegetables, and use a knife to make shallow cuts along the top so they don't split while heating. Transfer to the oven and cook for 20 minutes, or until the vegetables are tender and the sausages are browned.

While the sheet pan cooks, in a small bowl, combine the Buffalo sauce and ranch dressing and whisk together.

Serve the sausage and vegetables with a drizzle of Buffalo ranch and fresh chopped parsley to garnish.

QUICK TIP: Looking to cut back on time even more? Grab a bag of precut Brussels sprouts or sweet potatoes. A few minutes saved here and there can really add up!

COMBINATION PIZZA SKILLET

Nothing beats a pizza dinner until you realize you've spent $50 and have a stomachache. Is it worth it? Sometimes. But when you can satisfy all of those pizza cravings at home in under 30 minutes, and skip all of the gluten and dairy without even missing it? Now that's a win! Combination style is my favorite, but this easy skillet is ready to be fixed up however you love your pizza! It's truly all about the toppings—so make sure to pick your favorites.

YIELD: 4 SERVINGS
PREP TIME: 5 MINUTES
COOKING TIME: 19 MINUTES

1 lb (454 g) sweet Italian sausage

2 oz (57 g) pepperoni slices

1 medium green bell pepper, thinly sliced

½ medium red onion, thinly sliced

1 (2.25-oz [63-g]) can sliced black olives, drained

2 tsp (4 g) minced garlic

½ tsp dried Italian herb seasoning

¼ tsp red pepper flakes

¼ tsp oregano

¼ tsp salt

¼ tsp black pepper

1 (32-oz [900-g]) jar marinara sauce

Chopped fresh basil and red pepper flakes, for garnish

Heat a skillet over medium to medium-high and add the Italian sausage. Cook for 5 to 7 minutes, or until crumbled and browned. Add the pepperoni slices, bell pepper and red onion and cook for 4 to 5 minutes, or until the vegetables are tender. Stir in the sliced olives, garlic, Italian herb seasoning, red pepper flakes, oregano, salt, pepper and marinara sauce. Continue to cook, stirring occasionally, for 5 to 7 minutes, or until the sauce is warmed through.

Serve hot, garnished with fresh basil and red pepper flakes.

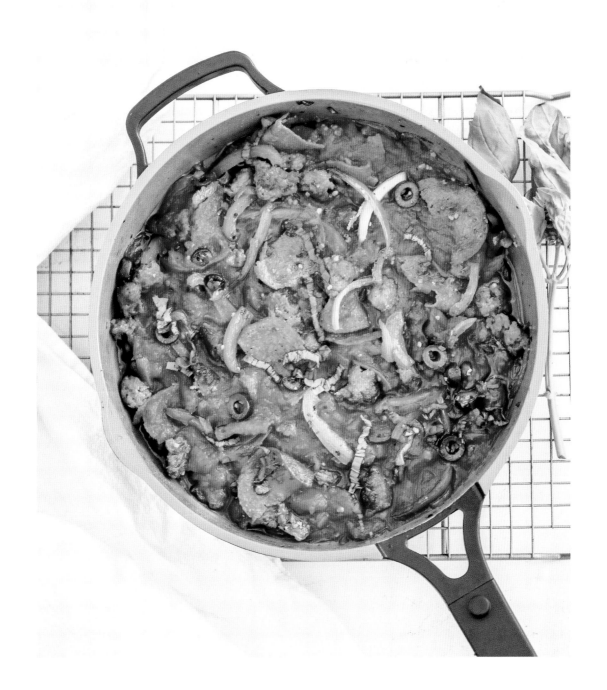

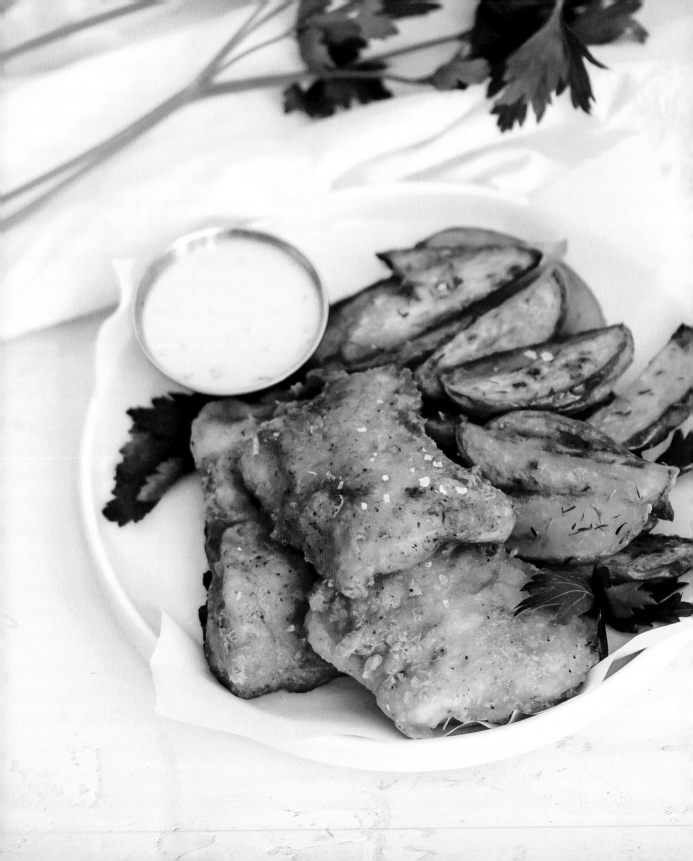

SEAFOOD IN A SNAP

Salmon, shrimp, mahi-mahi, oh my! From tacos to risotto to (fully cooked!) sushi bowls, I've got all of your seafood favorites covered in this chapter. Seafood is great for quick weeknight meals since it cooks so fast, but you don't want it overdone either! From the oven to the stovetop, I'll share my favorite methods for perfectly done fish and shrimp every time—with sauces and sides that will keep everyone asking for more.

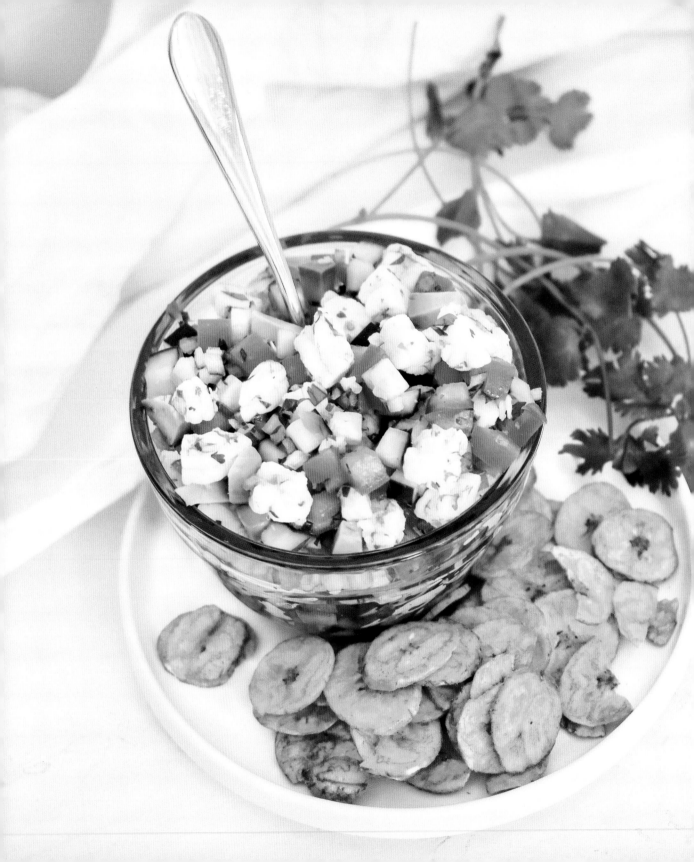

SPEEDY SHRIMP CEVICHE WITH AVOCADO

With this fresh and flavorful shrimp ceviche, we skip the long marinade time by cooking the shrimp first. It's a little shortcut that won't sacrifice any flavor—still tons of fresh lime, cilantro, chopped veggies and some cool, creamy avocado to bulk things up a bit. Serve it salad style over greens (it makes a great meal prep for lunches!) or traditional style with plantain or grain-free tortilla chips for some crunch.

YIELD: 8 CUPS (1.9 L)
PREP TIME: 20 MINUTES
COOKING TIME: 3 MINUTES

2 quarts (1.9 L) water

2 tsp (12 g) salt, divided

1 lb (454 g) raw shrimp, peeled and deveined

1 cup peeled, diced cucumber, ¼-inch (6-mm) dice

1 cup diced tomatoes, ¼-inch (6-mm) dice

½ cup (80 g) finely diced red onion

½ jalapeño pepper, seeded and minced

2 tbsp (2 g) chopped cilantro

Zest of 1 lime

Juice of 4 limes

1 large avocado, diced

Chopped romaine lettuce, plantain chips or tortilla chips, for serving

In a medium saucepan, bring the water and 1½ teaspoons (9 g) of salt to a boil. Turn off the heat and add the shrimp. Allow them to cook until opaque, 2 to 3 minutes. Immediately transfer the shrimp to a colander and rinse with cold water until cool.

Chop the cooked shrimp into ½-inch (1.3-cm) pieces. Place them in a large bowl and add the cucumber, tomatoes, red onion, jalapeño, cilantro, lime zest, lime juice and remaining ½ teaspoon of salt. If serving right away, add the avocado. If making ahead, keep the avocado whole and wait until just before serving to dice and stir in (so it doesn't brown).

Serve chilled over chopped romaine lettuce, or as a dip with plantain chips or grain-free tortilla chips.

QUICK TIP: To skip the cook time altogether, grab some fully cooked shrimp to use in this recipe!

THAI GREEN COCONUT CURRY WITH SHRIMP

Green curry is my favorite kind of curry—it's light, fresh, and has this great bright flavor from lemongrass and lime. I love sneaking in a jarred curry paste in so many of my recipes, as they pack in all of those traditional flavors in a fraction of the time. This one is topped with toasted cashews for some nutty crunch, and is perfect all on its own or served over your favorite rice!

YIELD: 4 SERVINGS
PREP TIME: 5 MINUTES
COOKING TIME: 14 MINUTES

1 tbsp (15 g) coconut oil

1 red bell pepper, sliced thin

1 medium white onion, diced

3 cloves garlic, minced

1 tsp minced ginger

3 tbsp (45 g) green curry paste

1 (14-oz [396-g]) can coconut milk

1 lb (454 g) shrimp, peeled and deveined

1 cup (30 g) packed baby spinach

½ cup (73 g) raw cashews

Cooked cauliflower rice, for serving (optional)

Chopped cilantro and lime wedges, for garnish

Heat the coconut oil in a skillet over medium heat. Add the bell pepper, onion, garlic and ginger and cook for 5 minutes, or until tender-crisp. Stir in the curry paste and coconut milk. Add the shrimp and baby spinach and bring to a simmer. Cover with a lid and cook for 3 to 4 minutes, or until the shrimp are just opaque.

To a separate dry pan, add the cashews and heat over medium-low, stirring occasionally, for about 5 minutes, or until golden and toasted.

Serve the curry alone or over cauliflower rice, topped with the toasted cashews, chopped cilantro and a squeeze of fresh lime juice.

QUICK TIP: Jarred curry pastes are such an easy way to add tons of traditional flavor with simple ingredients—all ready to go in your pantry.

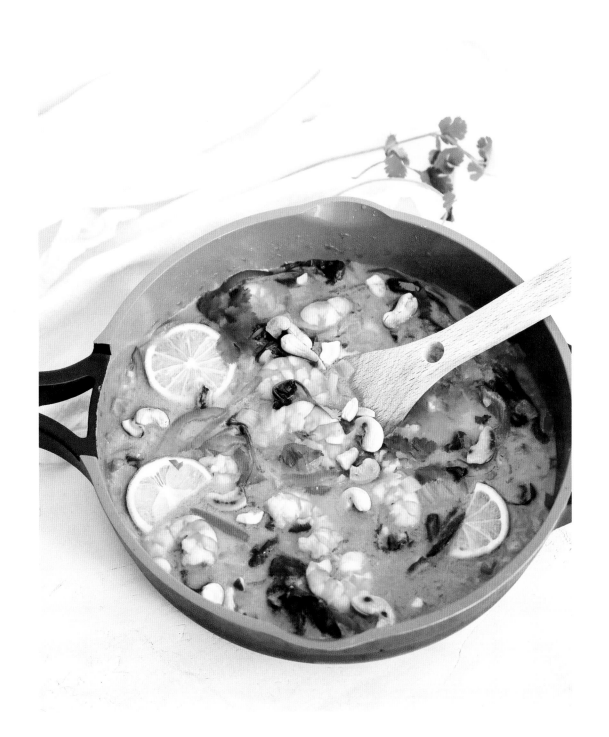

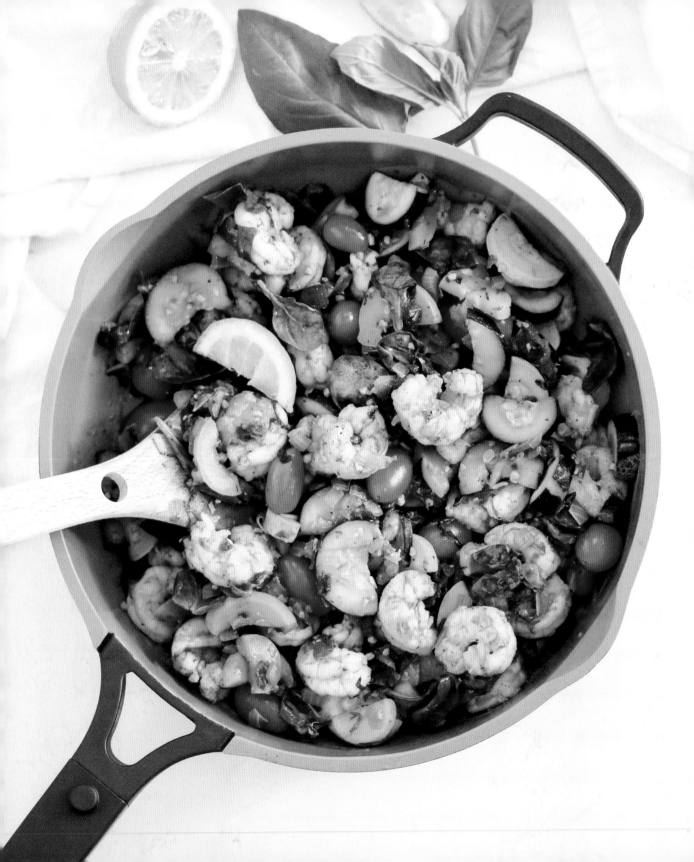

TUSCAN SHRIMP WITH GARDEN VEGETABLES

Garlic, Italian herbs and sun-dried tomatoes are a trio made in heaven, and they complement this shrimp and fresh vegetable skillet in the most perfect way. Add a squeeze of fresh lemon, and you'll feel like you've been whisked away to Tuscany in one bite! This dish is great on its own, but can also be served over smashed potatoes if you want to bulk things up.

YIELD: 4 SERVINGS
PREP TIME: 5 MINUTES
COOKING TIME: 13 MINUTES

1 tbsp (15 ml) olive oil

1 medium zucchini, halved lengthwise and sliced ¼ inch (6 mm) thick

1 yellow squash, halved lengthwise and sliced ¼ inch (6 mm) thick

½ medium yellow onion, diced

2 tsp (4 g) minced garlic

1 lb (454 g) shrimp, peeled and deveined

¼ cup (14 g) sun-dried tomatoes, julienned

½ tsp salt

½ tsp black pepper

½ tsp dried Italian herb seasoning

1 cup (30 g) baby spinach

1 cup (149 g) cherry tomatoes

2 tbsp (3 g) fresh basil, chopped

Lemon wedges, for garnish

In a skillet over medium to medium-high heat, heat the olive oil. Add the zucchini, squash, onion and garlic and sauté for 5 to 7 minutes, or until crisp tender. Add the shrimp, sun-dried tomatoes, salt, pepper and Italian herb seasoning and continue to sauté for 3 to 4 minutes, or until the shrimp is opaque. Stir in the spinach, cherry tomatoes and basil and cook for 2 more minutes, or until the spinach is wilted and the tomatoes are warm.

Serve hot or chilled leftover with fresh lemon wedges to garnish.

QUICK TIP: Jarred sun-dried tomatoes take this dish to the next level with a depth of flavor that takes time to establish, brought to you in seconds out of a glass jar. Look for the fewest ingredients with no added sulfites.

TERIYAKI-GLAZED SHRIMP & BROCCOLI SHEET PAN

Shrimp and broccoli are cooked to perfection on a single sheet pan in this simple yet tasty teriyaki dinner. The sticky teriyaki-style glaze is to die for and couldn't be easier—just simmer a few pantry-friendly ingredients on the stovetop while the sheet pan is in the oven, and you'll have a healthy dinner done in no time. Eat this alone or served over cauliflower rice (or white rice if your family does grains!) for a quick and delicious crowd-pleaser.

YIELD: 4 SERVINGS
PREP TIME: 5 MINUTES
COOKING TIME: 20 MINUTES

3 cups (270 g) broccoli florets

Avocado oil spray

1 lb (454 g) shrimp, peeled and deveined

½ tsp salt

½ cup (120 ml) coconut aminos

2 tbsp (30 ml) balsamic vinegar

1 tsp minced garlic

1 tbsp (15 ml) toasted sesame oil

1 tsp Dijon mustard

½ tsp minced ginger

¼ tsp red pepper flakes

1 tsp arrowroot powder mixed with 1 tbsp (15 ml) water (optional)

Sliced scallions and toasted sesame seeds, for garnish

Preheat the oven to 400°F (204°C). Line a baking sheet with parchment paper and arrange the broccoli florets in a single layer. Spray with avocado oil spray and transfer to the oven. Bake for 10 minutes.

Remove the sheet pan from the oven and add the shrimp, nestled between the broccoli florets. Season the entire dish with salt, and return to the oven for an additional 10 minutes.

While the shrimp and broccoli cook, make the teriyaki glaze. In a medium saucepan over medium-high heat, combine the coconut aminos, balsamic, garlic, sesame oil, Dijon mustard, ginger and red pepper flakes. Bring to a low boil, then reduce to a simmer. Cook, stirring frequently, until thickened enough to coat the back of a spoon, or about 5 minutes. If you like an even thicker glaze, combine the arrowroot and water in a small bowl to make a slurry. Stir in the arrowroot mixture (if using) and warm the sauce.

Serve the shrimp and broccoli with the teriyaki glaze poured over top, and garnish with scallions and toasted sesame seeds.

QUICK TIP: My favorite kind of balsamic is a nice thick one—even a reduction or glaze. It really adds flavor and cuts down on the amount of time it takes the sauce to thicken.

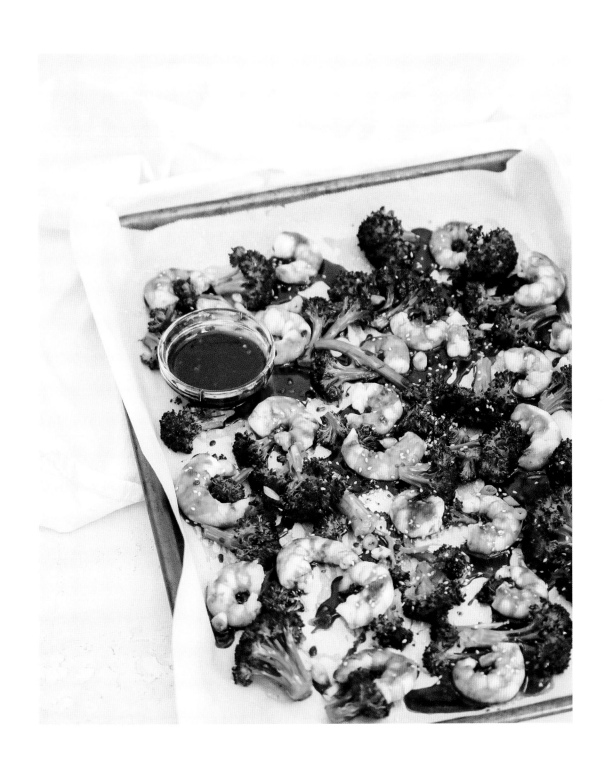

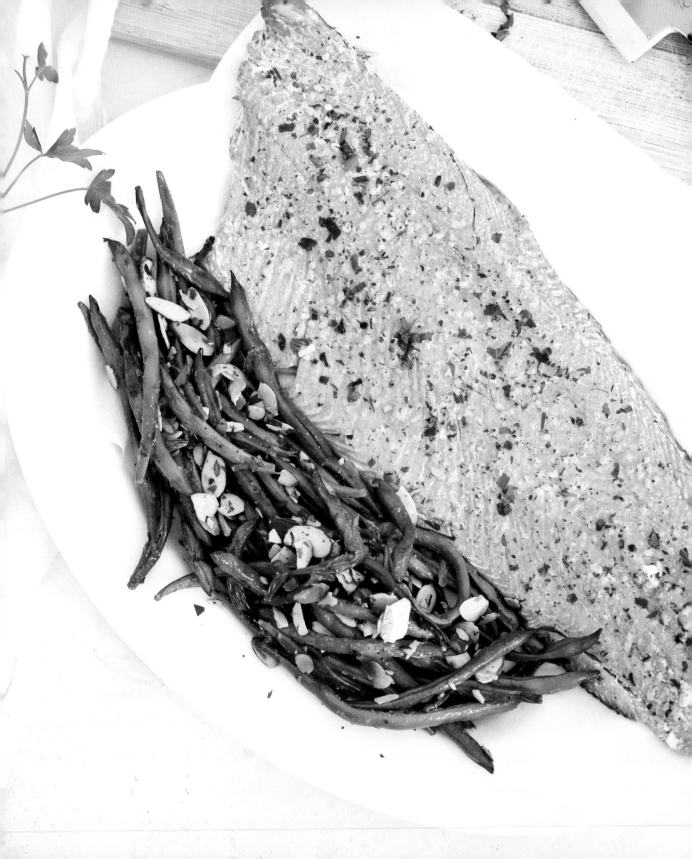

GARLIC BUTTER BAKED SALMON WITH GREEN BEANS ALMONDINE

Buttery broiled salmon with extra garlic is a go-to around here, mostly because it takes less than 10 minutes to make! But my favorite way to serve it up is with these perfect, savory "green beans almondine"—a nostalgic dish for me that my grandma loved. A woman after my own heart—because why have plain green beans when you can enjoy them sautéed in butter and mixed with warm, toasted almonds?

YIELD: 6 SERVINGS
PREP TIME: 10 MINUTES
COOKING TIME: 11 MINUTES

FOR THE SALMON

Avocado oil spray

1½ lb (681 g) whole salmon fillet

6 tbsp (90 g) ghee

2 tsp (4 g) minced garlic

½ tsp garlic powder

½ tsp dried parsley

½ tsp salt

¼ tsp red pepper flakes

FOR THE GREEN BEANS

3 tbsp (45 g) grass-fed butter or ghee, divided

½ cup (73 g) raw sliced almonds

1 lb (454 g) green beans, trimmed (thin are best)

1 tbsp (15 ml) water

½ tsp salt

½ tsp black pepper

½ tsp onion powder

To make the salmon: Set an oven rack in the uppermost position and preheat the oven to 400°F (204°C). Lightly coat a rimmed baking sheet with avocado oil spray. Place the salmon fillet on the greased baking sheet and pat the top dry with a paper towel. In a medium bowl, combine the ghee, minced garlic, garlic powder and dried parsley and microwave for 10 seconds at a time, until just softened (about 30 seconds total). Stir to combine, then use a butter knife or small rubber spatula to spread the mixture in an even layer over top of the salmon fillet. Season the whole fillet with salt and red pepper flakes. Transfer to the oven, and set it to broil. Cook for 6 to 8 minutes, or until the salmon flakes easily with a fork and is cooked through.

To make the green beans: While the salmon cooks, start on the green beans. Melt 1 tablespoon (15 g) of butter in a medium skillet over medium heat. Add the almonds to the pan and cook for 3 to 4 minutes, or until golden brown, stirring occasionally. Remove the almonds from the pan and wipe the pan clean with a paper towel.

Melt the remaining 2 tablespoons (30 g) of butter in the pan. Add the green beans and water to the pan. Cook, stirring occasionally, until the green beans are tender, about 5 minutes. Add the almonds back to the pan along with the salt, pepper and onion powder. Stir to combine and cook for 2 minutes to warm through.

Serve the salmon and green beans hot and enjoy!

GLAZED SALMON SUSHI BOWLS

If you are a sushi lover like me, but don't always have easy access to sushi-grade fish to serve up raw, this is for you! These bowls bring all of the fresh-meets-umami goodness that a great sushi roll does, but are served up bowl style with fully cooked salmon and an "unagi sauce"–style glaze.

YIELD: 4 SUSHI BOWLS
PREP TIME: 5 MINUTES
COOKING TIME: 13 MINUTES

4 salmon fillets

¼ cup (60 ml) coconut aminos

1 tsp minced ginger

1 tsp honey

2 tbsp (30 g) coconut oil, divided

12 oz (340 g) cauliflower rice

1 sheet sushi nori (roasted seaweed)

1 cup spring mix

1 medium cucumber, cut into ¼-inch (6-mm) dice or sliced thin

1 large avocado, sliced

Toasted sesame seeds, for garnish

Use a paper towel to pat the salmon fillets dry. In a large shallow bowl, whisk the coconut aminos, ginger and honey with a fork to combine. Add the salmon fillets to the glaze mixture. In a large skillet over medium-high heat, heat 1 tablespoon (15 g) of the coconut oil. Add the salmon to the hot pan, skin side down, leaving any extra glaze behind in the bowl. Cook for 5 minutes, or until a crust forms on the skin. Flip the salmon and cook for an additional 4 to 5 minutes, or until the fish is opaque and flakes easily with a fork. Remove the salmon from the pan, and add the glaze mixture to the hot pan. Bring to a simmer and cook for 2 to 3 minutes, or until just thickened. Reserve for topping the bowls when serving.

While the salmon cooks, in a medium saucepan over high heat, heat the remaining 1 tablespoon (15 g) of coconut oil. Add the cauliflower rice and cook for 2 to 3 minutes, or until just tender.

Slice the sushi nori thin, then roughly chop into small pieces.

To serve, divide the spring mix and cauliflower rice among four bowls. To each bowl, add one fillet of salmon, one-quarter of the cucumber, one-quarter of the sliced avocado and a handful of chopped nori. Drizzle the bowls with the thickened glaze and garnish with toasted sesame seeds.

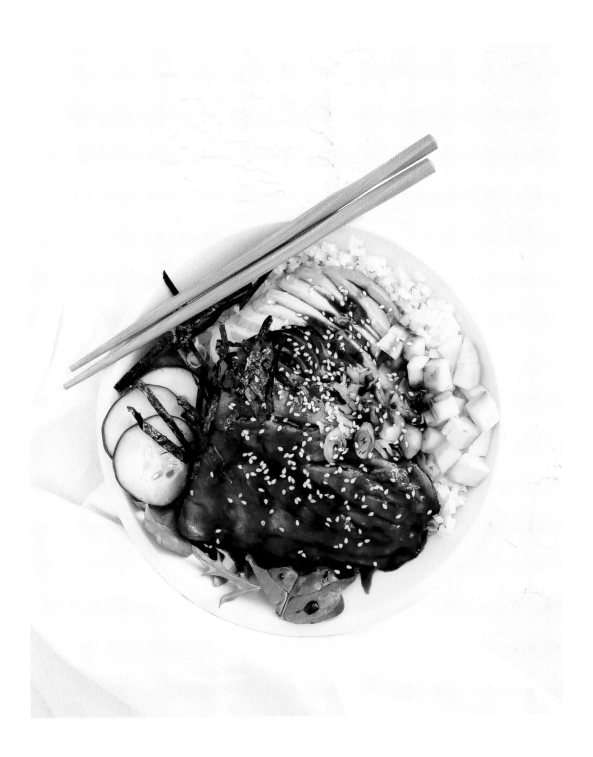

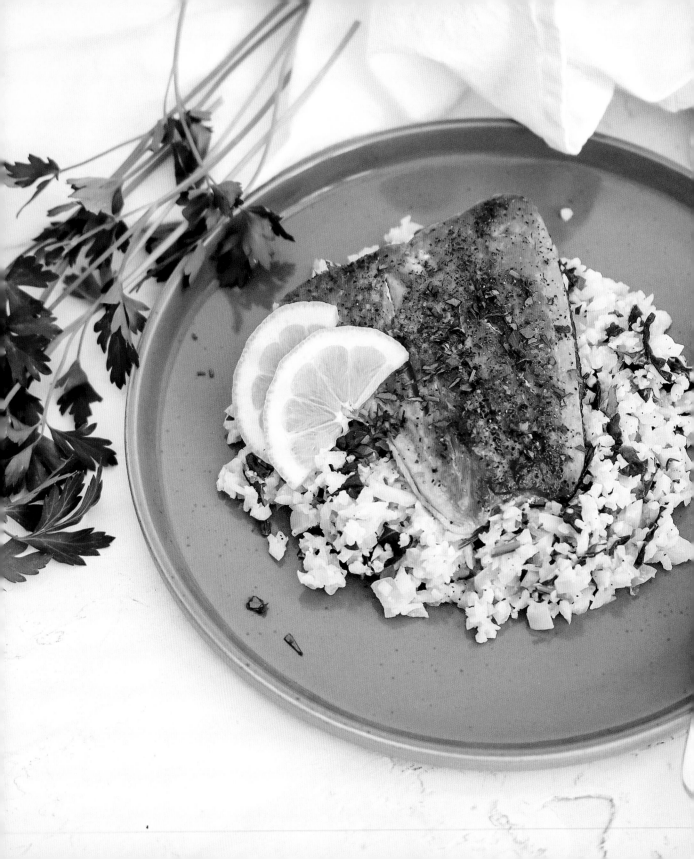

SEARED SALMON WITH CREAMY LEMON & SPINACH "RISOTTO"

Sometimes the simplest of dishes feel the most refined, and that is certainly the case for this one! Salt and pepper salmon is seared to perfection while a quick, creamy risotto comes together in just minutes. The key to making the cauliflower irresistible? Plenty of creaminess, and lots of bright, fresh lemon!

YIELD: 4 SERVINGS
PREP TIME: 5 MINUTES
COOKING TIME: 20 MINUTES

4 salmon fillets

1 tsp salt

1 tsp black pepper

1 tbsp (15 ml) olive oil

1 tbsp (15 g) ghee

½ medium yellow onion, diced

2 tsp (4 g) minced garlic

4 cups (960 ml) cauliflower rice

2 cups (60 g) baby spinach, chopped

½ cup (120 ml) dairy-free milk or cream

¼ cup (20 g) nutritional yeast

Zest of 1 lemon

Juice of 1 lemon

½ tsp salt

½ tsp black pepper

Chopped fresh parsley, for garnish

Lay the salmon fillets out on a cutting board and pat them dry with a paper towel. Season with salt and pepper. In a large skillet over medium-high heat, heat the olive oil. Add the salmon to the hot pan, skin side down. Cook for 5 minutes, or until a crust forms on the skin. Flip the salmon and cook for an additional 4 to 5 minutes, or until the fish is opaque and flakes easily with a fork.

While the salmon cooks, start the risotto. Melt the ghee in a saucepan over medium heat. Add the onion and garlic and sauté for about 2 minutes to soften. Turn the heat up to medium-high and add the cauliflower rice. Sauté for 3 minutes, or until just tender. Stir in the chopped spinach, milk, nutritional yeast, lemon zest, lemon juice, salt and pepper. Continue to cook until the milk is absorbed and the cauliflower is fluffy and creamy, 4 to 5 minutes.

Serve the salmon over the risotto and top with chopped fresh parsley.

QUICK TIP: I typically purchase boxed, shelf-stable coconut milk and dairy-free coffee creamers that I can keep on hand in the pantry. Either one works great for this recipe; the thicker and creamier, the better!

FIESTA FISH TACOS WITH SWEET CILANTRO-LIME SLAW

Make it a Taco Tuesday any day of the week with the ultimate fish tacos! In this recipe, white fish is baked to flaky perfection while you toss together a quick sweet lime slaw. Don't forget the crema—it balances out the acidity from the slaw and the heat from the fish just perfectly! Char up your favorite tortillas and enjoy!

YIELD: 8 TACOS
PREP TIME: 5 MINUTES
COOKING TIME: 22 MINUTES

FOR THE FISH

1½ lb (681 g) tilapia or cod
1 tsp chili powder
1 tsp cumin
1 tsp salt
¼ tsp cayenne (increase to ½ tsp if you like spice)
1 tbsp (15 ml) avocado oil

FOR THE CREMA

½ cup (120 ml) Paleo-friendly mayo
Juice of 1 lime
1 tsp garlic powder
1 tsp hot sauce

FOR THE SLAW

Juice of 1 lime
1 tbsp (15 ml) honey
2 tsp (10 ml) avocado oil
½ jalapeño pepper, thinly sliced
1 (16-oz [454-g]) bag coleslaw mix

FOR SERVING

8 grain-free tortillas
Chopped cilantro and fresh lime wedges, for garnish

To make the fish: Preheat the oven to 400°F (204°C). Line a baking sheet with parchment paper. Pat the fish dry with a paper towel, then lay it on the baking sheet. In a small bowl, combine the chili powder, cumin, salt and cayenne. Pat the seasoning onto both sides of the fish, then drizzle the avocado oil lightly over the top. Transfer to the oven and bake for 15 to 20 minutes, or until the fish is fully cooked and flakes easily with a fork.

To make the crema and slaw: While the fish cooks, prepare the crema and slaw. In a small bowl, combine the mayo, lime juice, garlic powder and hot sauce and stir until smooth. Transfer to the refrigerator until ready to serve.

In a large bowl, combine the lime juice, honey and avocado oil and whisk until combined. Add the sliced jalapeño and coleslaw mix and stir to coat with the dressing. Transfer to the refrigerator until the fish is done.

To serve: When the fish is done, use a fork to flake into chunks. To serve, char the tortillas over a low flame until lightly browned or warm them in a pan. Fill each tortilla halfway with slaw and top with fish and a drizzle of crema. Garnish with chopped cilantro and a squeeze of fresh lime.

QUICK TIP: Grain-free tortillas are becoming increasingly easy to find at most stores, and they freeze so well! I look for the cassava ones since they hold up well and don't crumble as easily as other varieties. Store them in the freezer, then thaw them overnight in the fridge or stick the whole pack in some warm water while you prep the rest of the meal—they defrost really quickly!

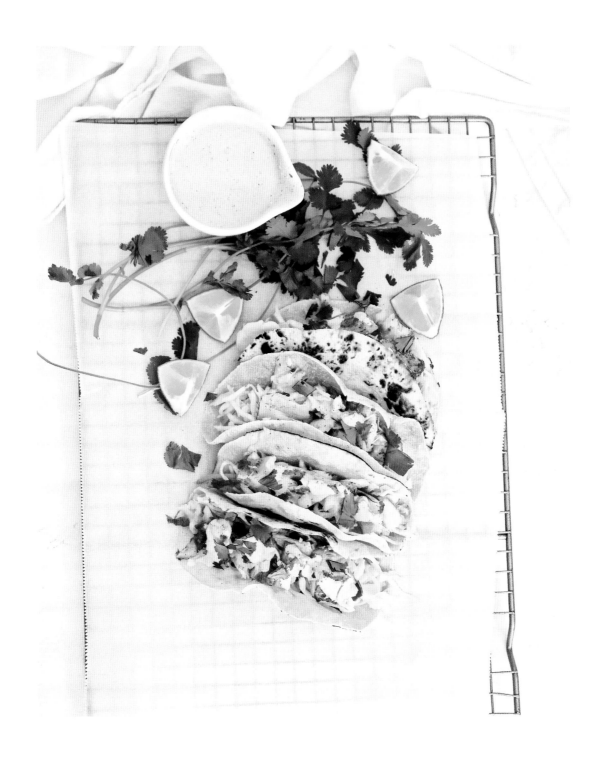

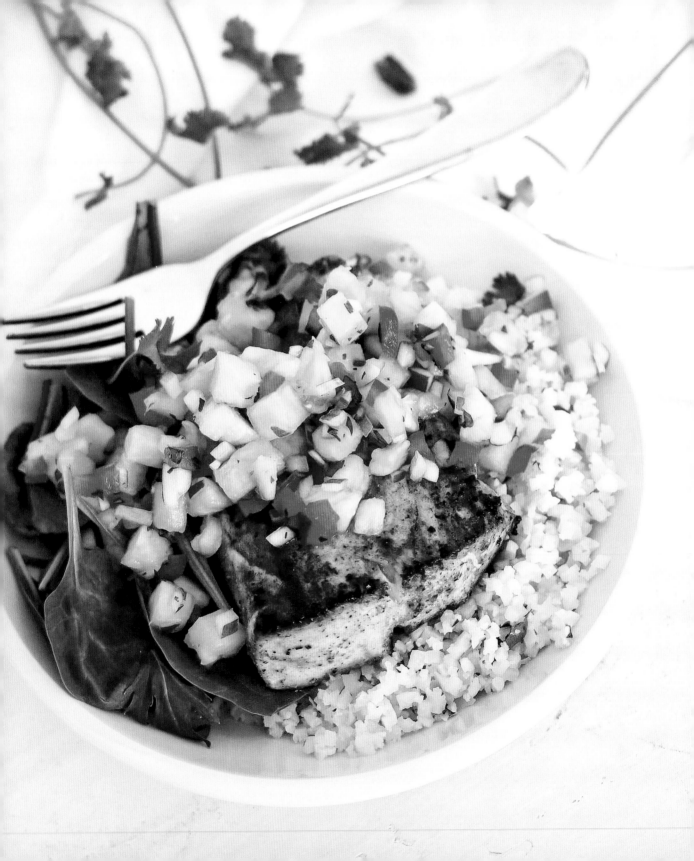

MAHI-MAHI RICE BOWLS WITH PINEAPPLE SALSA

There's something about pineapple salsa that adds the perfect sweet bite to a savory dish, without overpowering it. This one has red bell pepper mixed in for crunch and plenty of fresh lime juice to keep things bright. Serve it over tender, meaty mahi-mahi coated in a taco-style blend, and you'll feel like you're on "some beach, somewhere" . . . even if it's a regular Wednesday.

YIELD: 4 BOWLS
PREP TIME: 15 MINUTES
COOKING TIME: 14 MINUTES

FOR THE PINEAPPLE SALSA

3 cups (495 g) diced fresh pineapple (1 medium pineapple)

1 medium red bell pepper, chopped

1 small red onion, chopped

¼ cup (4 g) chopped cilantro

1 medium jalapeño, seeded and minced

3 tbsp (45 ml) lime juice

¼ tsp salt

FOR THE MAHI-MAHI

2 tbsp (30 ml) avocado oil

2 tbsp (30 ml) lime juice

1 tsp cumin

1 tsp chili powder

½ tsp smoked paprika

½ tsp garlic powder

½ tsp salt

½ tsp black pepper

4 mahi-mahi fillets

FOR THE CAULIFLOWER RICE

1 tsp avocado oil

12 oz (340 g) cauliflower rice

2 tbsp (2 g) chopped cilantro

1 tbsp (15 ml) lime juice

To make the pineapple salsa: In a medium bowl, combine the pineapple, bell pepper, onion, cilantro, jalapeño, lime juice and salt and cover. Transfer to the refrigerator and chill until ready to serve.

To make the mahi-mahi: In a dish large enough to fit the fish, combine the avocado oil, lime juice, cumin, chili powder, paprika, garlic, salt and pepper. Pat the mahi-mahi fillets dry with a paper towel. Add the fish to the spice mixture, allowing the marinade to fully coat each fillet on both sides. Heat a grill pan or large skillet to medium-high heat. Add the fish, and grill for 5 to 7 minutes on each side, or until opaque through the center.

To make the cauliflower rice: While the fish cooks, heat the avocado oil in a medium saucepan over high heat. Add the cauliflower rice and cook for 3 minutes, or until just tender. Turn off the heat and stir in the chopped cilantro and lime juice.

Serve in bowls with cauliflower rice, mahi-mahi and a scoop of pineapple salsa on top.

QUICK TIP: This recipe makes a large amount of the pineapple salsa, which can turn any quick weeknight meal special fast! Try it over grilled chicken, salmon, shrimp, any salad or even as a dip with plantain chips.

"FISH & CHIPS": CRISPY BATTERED FISH & OVEN FRIES

If you would have told me years ago, when I first started eating a Paleo diet, that I could have fish and chips that tasted like legitimate Monterey Bay restaurant-style fish and chips, crunchy fried batter and all, I would have never believed it! This recipe will fool even the pickiest of eaters—it's an absolute classic done grain free and cooked in a healthy oil, and so delicious you will come back to it again and again!

YIELD: 4 SERVINGS
PREP TIME: 10 MINUTES
COOKING TIME: 20 MINUTES

FOR THE OVEN FRIES

4 medium Yukon gold potatoes, cut into wedges ¼ inch (6 mm) thick or less

2 tbsp (30 ml) avocado oil

1 tsp salt

½ tsp dried thyme

FOR THE FISH

1 lb (454 g) white fish, such as cod or haddock

2 tsp (12 g) salt, plus more to taste

½ tsp black pepper

¾ cup (94 g) tapioca flour

2 eggs

1 tsp white vinegar

½ tsp baking soda

½ cup (120 ml) avocado oil, for frying

To make the oven fries: Preheat the oven to 450°F (232°C) and line a baking sheet with parchment paper (use two baking sheets if needed). In a large bowl, toss the potato wedges with oil, salt and thyme. Arrange them on the baking sheet in a single layer. Transfer to the oven and bake for 20 minutes total, flipping once halfway through.

To make the fish: While the potatoes are baking, lay the fish out on a cutting board and cut into fillets about 3 to 4 inches (7.5 to 10 cm) in length. Pat them dry with a paper towel and season with salt and pepper. In a large bowl, combine the tapioca flour, eggs, vinegar and baking soda and whisk until smooth. Add the seasoned fish to the bowl of batter.

Heat the avocado oil in a large pot or Dutch oven over medium heat. Add the fish to the hot oil in two separate batches to allow space, and fry for 3 minutes, or until golden brown. Carefully flip with a large spatula, and cook for an additional 5 minutes, or until an internal temperature reads 145°F (62°C) on an instant read thermometer and both sides are golden-brown. Transfer to a cooling rack lined with a paper towel while you cook the second batch. Season the cooked fish with additional salt to taste.

Serve the hot fish and chips together with a dipping sauce of your choice.

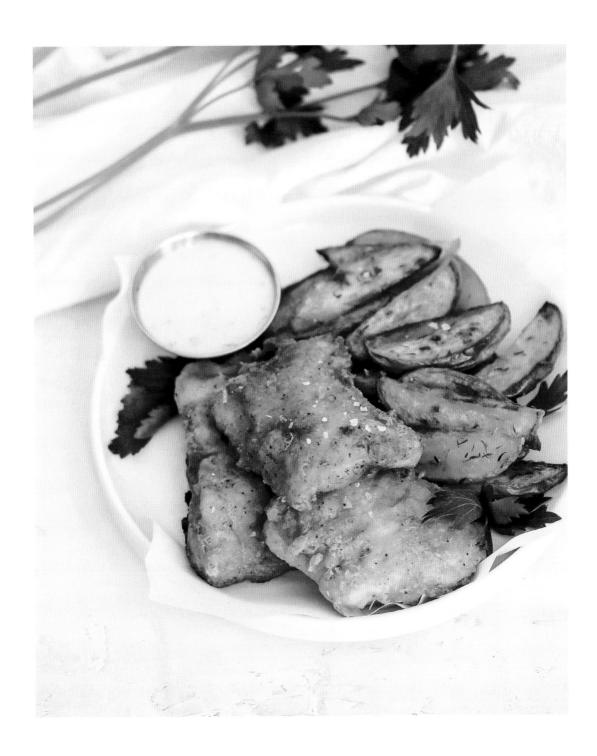

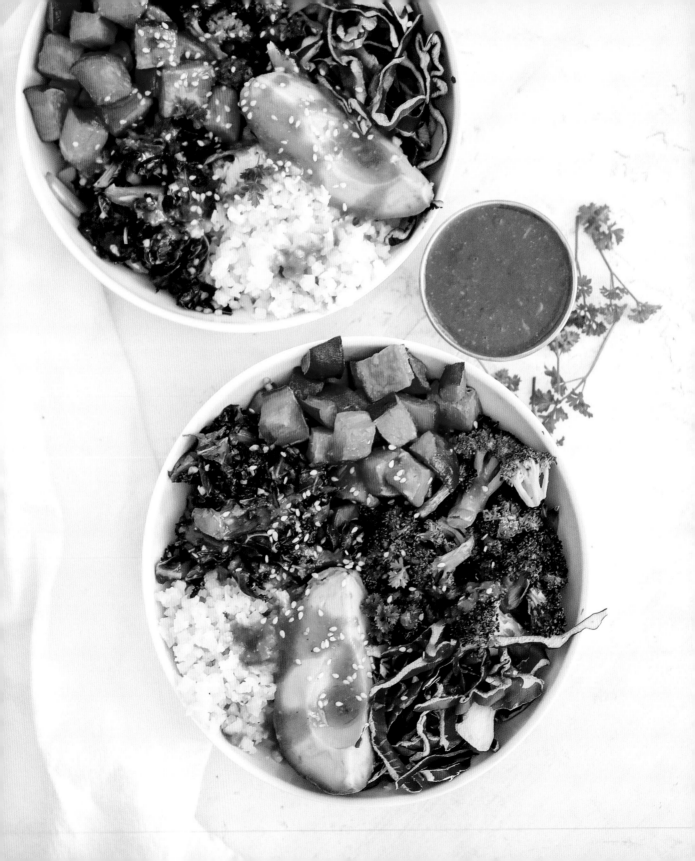

PLANT-BASED EXPRESS

Plant-based dishes are a great way to experiment with new foods and flavors, and are honestly . . . a challenge for me! While I typically find myself relying heavily on meats for balanced meals, this chapter will bring out the vegetarian in us all! Each dish is hearty, satisfying and full of delicious flavor. From comfort food classics to fun new flavors you may have never experienced before, I hope you'll enjoy these meals (and if you wanted to serve them up alongside a great protein of choice, I won't judge!). They all make for beautiful, filling side dishes, too!

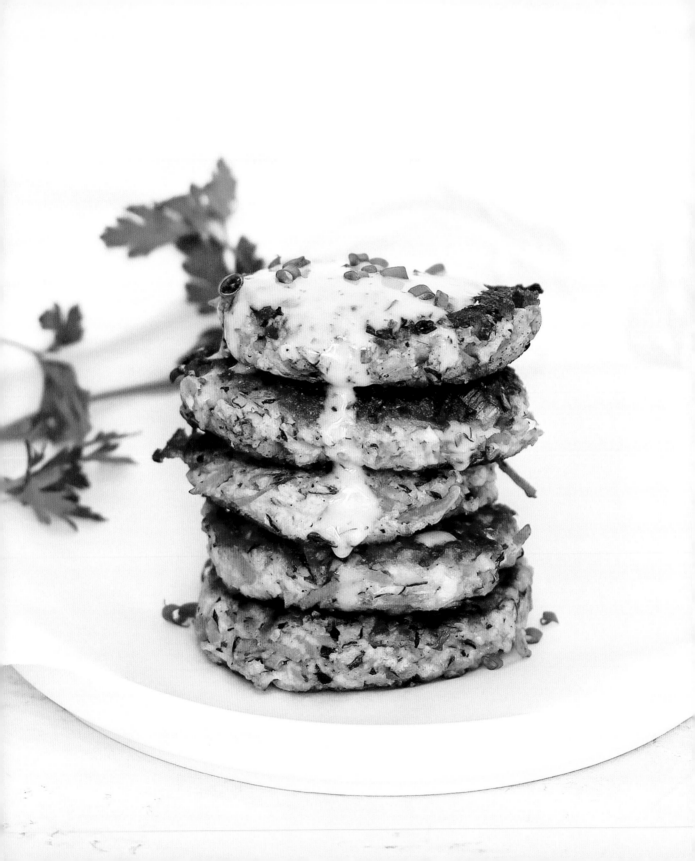

CRISPY CARROT & ZUCCHINI FRITTERS

Savory, crispy and veggie-packed, these fritters are the perfect kid-friendly dish that the grown-ups will love, too! Serve them up "burger bowl" style over greens with your favorite toppings, or keep it simple with some ranch to dip. The healthy fats from almonds and coconut oil make these super satisfying—but feel free to double the recipe if you're feeding a crowd!

YIELD: 7 FRITTERS
PREP TIME: 10 MINUTES
COOKING TIME: 6 MINUTES

2 medium zucchini

4 large carrots

⅔ cup (71 g) almond flour

2 large eggs

½ tsp garlic powder

½ tsp onion powder

½ tsp salt

½ tsp black pepper

⅓ cup (16 g) sliced scallion

2 tbsp (30 g) coconut oil

Paleo-friendly ranch dressing, for serving

Shred the zucchini and carrots using a cheese grater or a food processor with a shredding attachment. Wrap the veggies in cheesecloth or a double layer of paper towels and squeeze out as much moisture as you can. Transfer them to a bowl and add the almond flour, eggs, garlic powder, onion powder, salt, pepper and scallion. Mix with a large fork until combined. Use a ¼-cup (60-ml) measuring cup to scoop out portions of the mixture into your hands. Form each into a round patty shape about ½ to ¾ inch (1.3 to 2 cm) thick.

In a large skillet over medium to medium-high heat, heat the coconut oil. Add the fritters and cook for about 3 minutes per side, or until golden brown. Transfer to a cooling rack lined with a paper towel to absorb any excess oil.

Serve hot with Paleo-friendly ranch dressing.

QUICK TIP: I can always find pre-grated carrots at the store, and I'm all about saving a few minutes! I just make sure to give them a quick chop if needed, so they are smaller in size and easier to incorporate into the patties. 2 cups (220 g) of pre-grated carrots will work in place of shredding your own.

INDIAN EGGPLANT CURRY

Eggplant, or "aubergine," is one of my favorite vegetables for adding heartiness to plant-based dishes. When it's paired with full-fat coconut milk and lots of beautiful warm spices, and served over cauliflower rice, this dish will leave your belly full and your senses singing. You can easily adjust the level of heat in this recipe by adding more or less (or no) cayenne pepper. Don't forget the fresh lime and chopped cilantro to really bring your bowl to life!

YIELD: 4 SERVINGS
PREP TIME: 5 MINUTES
COOKING TIME: 12 MINUTES

1 tbsp (15 ml) olive oil

1 medium eggplant, quartered lengthwise then sliced into ½-inch (1.3-cm)-thick pieces

½ medium red onion, finely diced

3 cloves garlic, minced

1 (14.5-oz [428-ml]) can coconut milk

1 (14.5-oz [411-g]) can petite diced tomatoes

1 tsp curry powder

1 tsp turmeric

1 tsp coriander

½ tsp salt

⅛ tsp cayenne

4 cups (400 g) steamed cauliflower rice, for serving

1 lime, cut into wedges, for serving

½ cup (8 g) chopped cilantro, for garnish

In a large skillet over medium-high heat, heat the olive oil. Add the eggplant, onion and garlic and cook for 5 to 7 minutes, or until the eggplant is tender and lightly browned and the onion is soft. Add the coconut milk, diced tomatoes, curry powder, turmeric and coriander and stir to combine. Season with salt and cayenne, then taste to see if you'd like to add more. Simmer for 5 minutes, or until the coconut milk has thickened just enough to coat the back of a spoon.

Serve hot, scooped over 1 cup (100 g) of steamed cauliflower rice. Top with a squeeze of fresh lime and chopped cilantro to garnish.

QUICK TIP: This recipe is super hearty on its own, but also a great one to add chicken to if you have meat lovers in the group. Stir in some shredded rotisserie chicken for an easy protein addition!

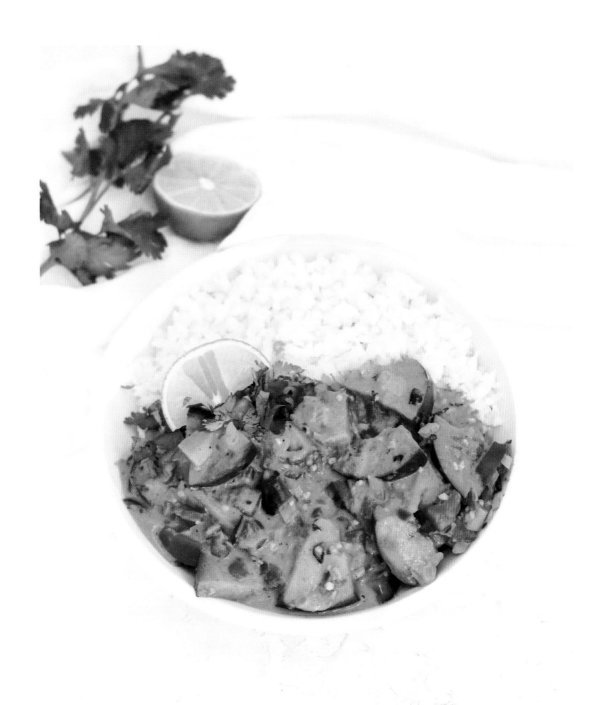

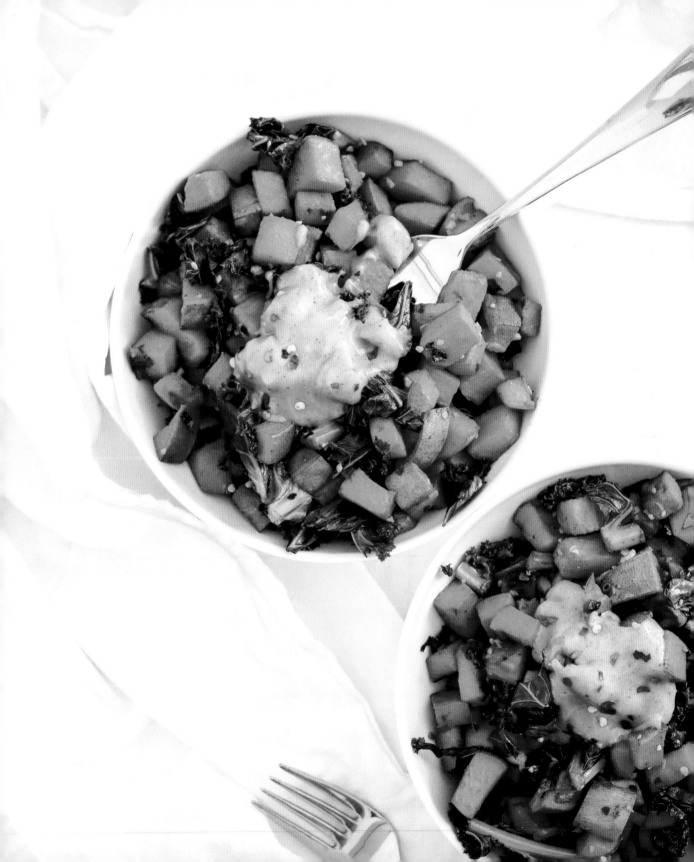

SAVORY SWEET POTATO & KALE HASH WITH MAPLE-TAHINI SAUCE

This dish is a balancing act when it comes to flavor: savory, sweet, spicy, warm—a little bitterness from the kale balanced just right by the sweetness of the sweet potato. Serve it up bowl style and top with a dollop of sweet, nutty maple-tahini sauce—try not to eat the whole pan! You will be amazed at how satisfying this bowl of veggie goodness can be.

YIELD: 6 CUPS (1.4 L)
PREP TIME: 5 MINUTES
COOKING TIME: 15 MINUTES

FOR THE HASH

1½ tbsp (22 ml) olive oil

3 medium sweet potatoes, cut into ½-inch (1.3-cm) cubes

½ tsp onion powder

½ tsp salt

½ tsp black pepper

¼ tsp cinnamon

¼ tsp red pepper flakes

4 loosely packed cups (268 g) chopped kale

3 cloves garlic, minced

FOR THE MAPLE-TAHINI SAUCE

⅓ cup (80 ml) tahini

1 tbsp (15 ml) maple syrup

½ tsp cinnamon

½ tsp smoked paprika

½ tsp apple cider vinegar

¼ tsp salt

2 tbsp (30 ml) water, plus more if needed

To make the hash: In a large skillet over medium to medium-high heat, heat the olive oil. Add the cubed sweet potatoes and cook for 10 minutes, stirring occasionally, until the potatoes are fork-tender. Stir in the onion powder, salt, pepper, cinnamon and red pepper flakes. Add the kale and garlic and continue to cook for 5 minutes, or until the kale is tender-crisp and garlic is softened.

To make the maple-tahini sauce: In a small bowl, combine the tahini, maple syrup, cinnamon, paprika, apple cider vinegar and salt and stir together. Add the water, 1 tablespoon (15 ml) at a time, until the sauce reaches your preferred consistency. I like it thin enough to drizzle but thick enough to coat the spoon.

Serve hot in bowls with a spoonful of maple-tahini sauce.

QUICK TIP: Pre-chopped kale with the big, thick stems removed is my favorite bagged vegetable to keep on hand. It adds the perfect texture and saves you the extra work of trimming and chopping!

VEGGIE BUDDHA BOWLS WITH SESAME DRIZZLE

A "Buddha bowl" is typically a one-bowl vegetarian meal full of several different foods served all together in smaller portions. This recipe marries the fresh, the roasted and the sautéed together for a variety of textures that will keep you coming back for bite after bite. When topped with my "peanut-style" sesame drizzle, this dish is so addicting, you'll forget you're eating a bowl full of veggies!

YIELD: 4 BOWLS
PREP TIME: 5 MINUTES
COOKING TIME: 20 TO 25 MINUTES

FOR THE BUDDHA BOWLS

2 medium sweet potatoes, cut into ½-inch (1.3-cm) cubes

3 cups (273 g) broccoli florets, broken into bite-sized pieces

2 tbsp (30 ml) avocado oil

2 tbsp (30 g) coconut oil, divided

2 cups (134 g) kale, chopped

2 tsp (4 g) minced garlic

4 cups (400 g) cauliflower rice

1 large avocado, sliced

1½ cups (105 g) shredded red cabbage

FOR THE SESAME DRIZZLE

½ cup (120 ml) tahini

¼ cup (65 g) creamy cashew butter

¼ cup (60 ml) coconut aminos

2 tbsp (30 ml) rice vinegar

¼ cup (60 ml) maple syrup

1 tsp minced ginger

1 tsp hot sauce

2–6 tbsp (30–90 ml) coconut milk, to thin

Toasted sesame seeds, for garnish

To make the vegetables: Preheat the oven to 425°F (218°C). Line a baking sheet with parchment paper and add the cubed sweet potatoes and broccoli florets in a single layer. Drizzle with the avocado oil and transfer to the oven. Bake for 20 to 25 minutes, or until the sweet potatoes are tender and the broccoli is crisp.

Heat 1 tablespoon (15 g) of coconut oil in a large skillet over medium heat. Add the kale and garlic and cook for 7 to 8 minutes, stirring occasionally, until tender.

Heat the remaining 1 tablespoon (15 g) of coconut oil in a medium saucepan over high heat. Add the cauliflower rice and sauté for 3 minutes, or until just tender.

To make the sesame drizzle: While the vegetables cook, make the drizzle in a small bowl by combining the tahini, cashew butter, coconut aminos, rice vinegar, maple syrup, ginger and hot sauce and whisking until smooth. Add the coconut milk, 1 tablespoon (15 ml) at a time, until it reaches a consistency you like—thin enough to drizzle.

Serve in four bowls with roasted vegetables, garlicky kale, cauliflower rice, avocado, cabbage and sesame drizzle. Garnish with toasted sesame seeds.

QUICK TIP: This drizzle deserves a permanent home in your refrigerator! Make a double batch and save in a lidded jar in the fridge for dressing up an Asian-style salad any time or dipping raw veggies. It's a lunch hour's best friend!

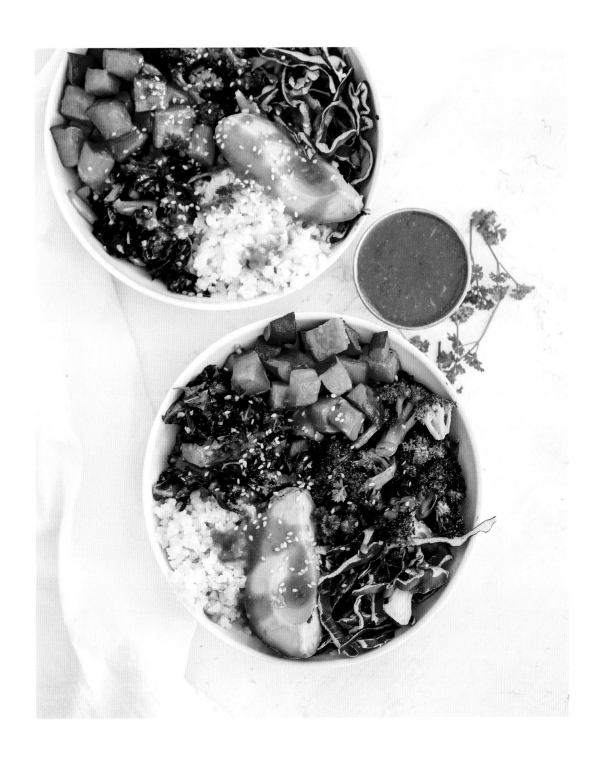

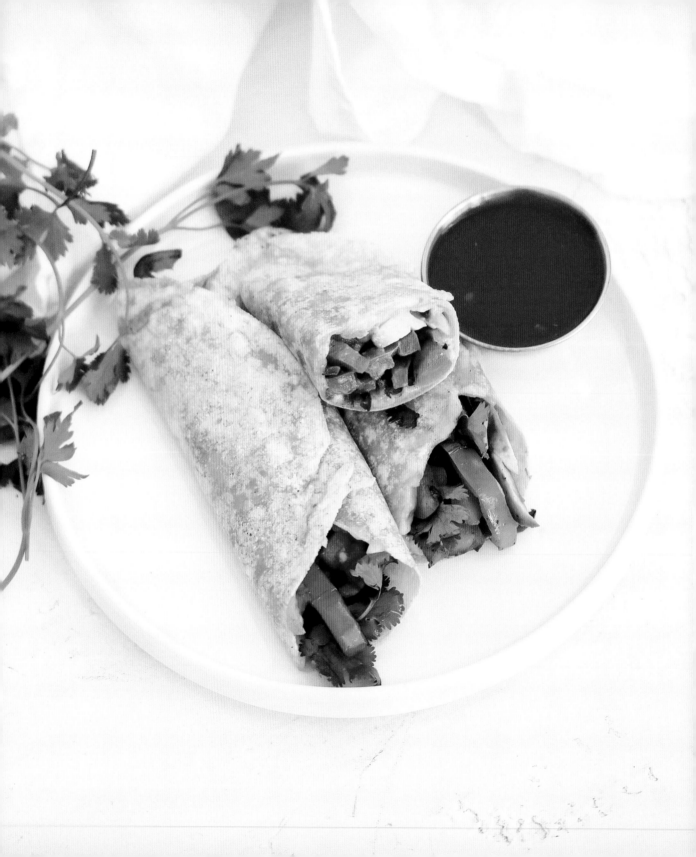

SKILLET VEGETABLE FAJITA BURRITOS

Burritos and Paleo may sound like they don't belong in the same sentence—especially if you add the phrase "plant-based" to that! But I'm here to defy all odds with the most delicious little veggie burritos. Tons of fajita flavor, all the fixings, and so satisfying!

YIELD: 4 BURRITOS
PREP TIME: 5 MINUTES
COOKING TIME: 12 MINUTES

1 tbsp (15 ml) avocado oil

1 green bell pepper, sliced

1 red bell pepper, sliced

1 small red onion, thinly sliced

½ tsp cumin

½ tsp chili powder

¼ tsp salt

¼ tsp oregano

4 grain-free tortillas

1 cup (112 g) dairy-free shredded cheese

½ cup (120 ml) pico de gallo

1 large avocado, sliced

In a medium skillet over medium-high heat, heat the avocado oil. Add the sliced bell peppers, onion, cumin, chili powder, salt and oregano, tossing to coat. Sauté for 4 to 5 minutes, or until the vegetables are tender and browned.

Heat a medium skillet over medium heat and lay 1 tortilla at a time in the warm, dry skillet. Sprinkle the tortilla with ¼ cup (28 g) of cheese and cover the skillet with a lid for 2 minutes, or until the cheese is melted. Transfer to a plate, and arrange one-fourth of the fajita vegetables in the center of the tortilla. Top with 2 tablespoons (30 ml) of pico de gallo and one-quarter of the avocado slices, then wrap up the tortilla, folding in the sides first. Repeat for the remaining tortillas to make four burritos.

QUICK TIP: To save these for a super-fast future meal, wrap the burritos in parchment paper or foil and then transfer them to the fridge. Reheat them in a microwave or air fryer when you're ready to enjoy!

HARVEST SWEET POTATO SHEET PAN WITH BRUSSELS & CRANBERRIES

If fall was a dish, this would be it! In fact, it's both delicious and beautiful enough that it will be gracing our Thanksgiving table for years to come. Sweet meets savory meets nutty and bright in this double sheet pan meal tossed with the most delicious dressing. Add an extra flair with dried cranberries (or cherries if you prefer!).

YIELD: 8 CUPS (1.9 L)
PREP TIME: 7 MINUTES
COOKING TIME: 20 MINUTES

1 lb (454 g) Brussels sprouts, halved

2 tsp (4 g) minced garlic

1 large sweet potato, cut into ½- to 1-inch (1.3- to 2.5-cm) cubes (about 4 cups)

⅓ cup (36 g) pecans

1 tsp salt, divided, plus more to taste

1 tsp black pepper, divided

Avocado or olive oil spray

1 tbsp (15 ml) olive oil

1 tbsp (15 ml) honey

2 tsp (10 ml) balsamic vinegar

⅓ cup (40 g) dried cranberries or cherries

Preheat the oven to 425°F (218°C). Line two baking sheets with parchment paper. To one baking sheet, add the Brussels sprouts and minced garlic. To the other baking sheet, add the sweet potato and pecans. Sprinkle ½ teaspoon of the salt and ½ teaspoon of the pepper over both baking sheets, then spray each with a light coating of avocado oil spray. Transfer both baking sheets to the oven and bake for 20 minutes, or until the vegetables are tender and light golden brown.

Whisk the olive oil, honey and balsamic in the bottom of a serving bowl large enough to fit the entire 8 cups (1.9 L) of the recipe. When the vegetables are done cooking, add them to the large bowl along with the dried cranberries or cherries, and toss to combine.

Serve warm, with additional salt to taste.

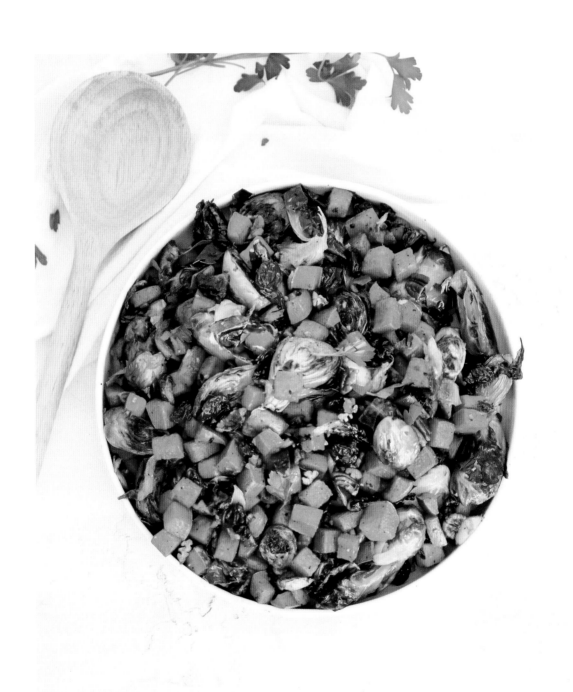

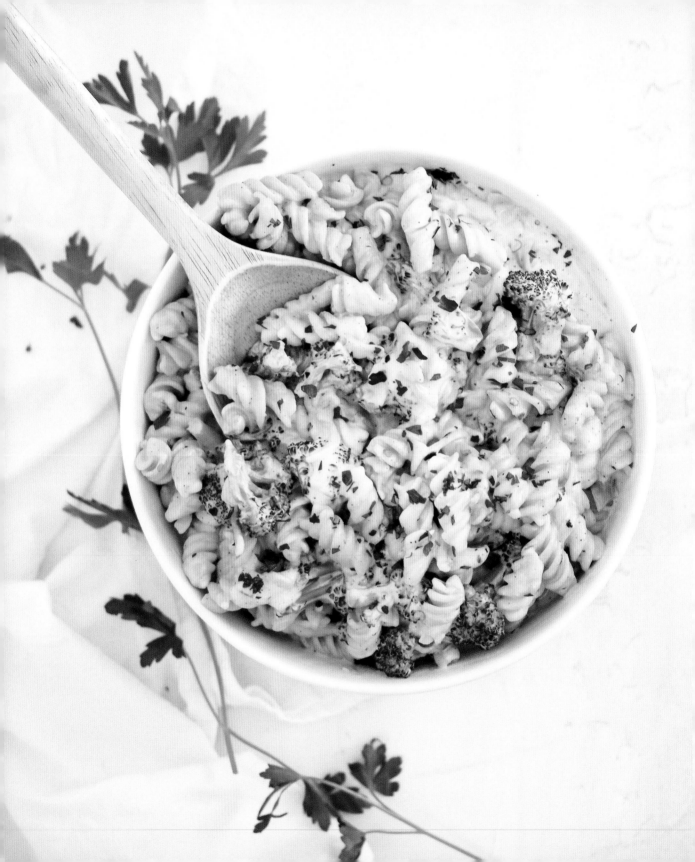

GARLICKY ALFREDO PASTA WITH BROCCOLI & SPINACH

Everyone has their ultimate comfort food, and this Alfredo is mine. My mom always added broccoli to ours, and I love how simple it is to add an extra veggie with no extra dishes and minimal effort. And speaking of minimal effort, this Alfredo sauce is as easy as they come and one of my favorites of all time. I promise you it is just as good as (honestly better than) the real deal!

YIELD: 8 CUPS (1.6 KG) OF PASTA
PREP TIME: 10 MINUTES
COOKING TIME: 15 MINUTES

1 lb (454 g) Paleo-friendly pasta (I use rotini)

2 cups (182 g) broccoli florets, broken into small pieces

1 cup (146 g) raw cashews

1 cup (240 ml) coconut milk

1 cup (240 ml) vegetable broth

¼ cup (20 g) nutritional yeast

2 tbsp (30 g) ghee or olive oil

2 tsp (5 g) garlic powder

1 tsp onion powder

1 tsp salt

½ tsp black pepper

1 tsp dried Italian herb seasoning

¼ tsp red pepper flakes, plus more to taste

Cook the pasta in a large pot according to package instructions, until al dente. During the last 2 minutes of cook time, add the broccoli and continue to boil. Drain the pasta and broccoli, then return them to the pot.

While the pasta cooks, in a high-speed blender or food processor, combine the cashews, coconut milk, vegetable broth, nutritional yeast, ghee, garlic powder, onion powder, salt and pepper. Pulse until super smooth, 1 to 2 minutes.

Add the Alfredo sauce to the pasta and broccoli along with the Italian herb seasoning and red pepper flakes and stir to combine. Serve hot!

QUICK TIP: Double the recipe for the Alfredo sauce and keep a jar of it in the refrigerator for another easy meal! Use the sauce within 1 week.

ROASTED CAULIFLOWER "MAC & CHEESE"

Just trust me when I tell you you're not going to miss the cheese here! This sauce is creamy, savory, smooth and even stretches like the real deal. It is so good, and makes eating a bowl full of cauliflower an easy task (even for the picky ones!). You'll want to double this recipe, because you'll be going back for seconds!

YIELD: 4 CUPS (920 G)
PREP TIME: 5 MINUTES
COOKING TIME: 20 TO 25 MINUTES

1 large head cauliflower, cut into florets and broken into small pieces

1 tbsp (15 ml) olive oil

1 tbsp (15 g) ghee

2 tbsp (16 g) tapioca flour

1 cup (240 ml) coconut milk

¼ cup (20 g) nutritional yeast

½ tsp salt

½ tsp garlic powder

½ tsp onion powder

¼ tsp smoked paprika

Finely chopped parsley, for garnish

Preheat the oven to 400°F (204°C). Line a baking sheet with parchment paper, and arrange the cauliflower pieces in a single layer. Drizzle with the olive oil and transfer to the oven. Bake for 20 to 25 minutes, or until the cauliflower is tender and browned.

While the cauliflower cooks, make the sauce. In a medium saucepan over medium-low heat, melt the ghee. Add the tapioca flour and stir to combine. Stir in the coconut milk, nutritional yeast, salt, garlic powder, onion powder and smoked paprika. Simmer until warm and stretchy, stirring continuously, about 2 minutes.

Add the roasted cauliflower to the sauce and stir to coat. Serve hot with chopped fresh parsley to garnish.

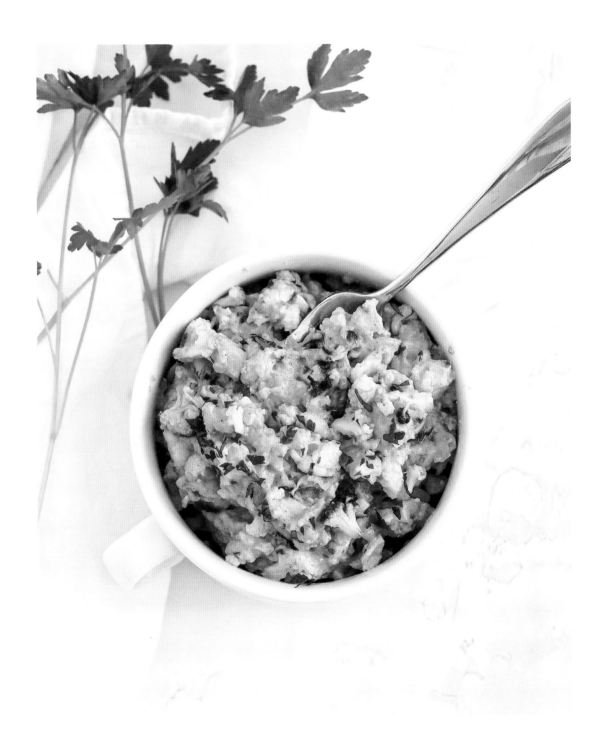

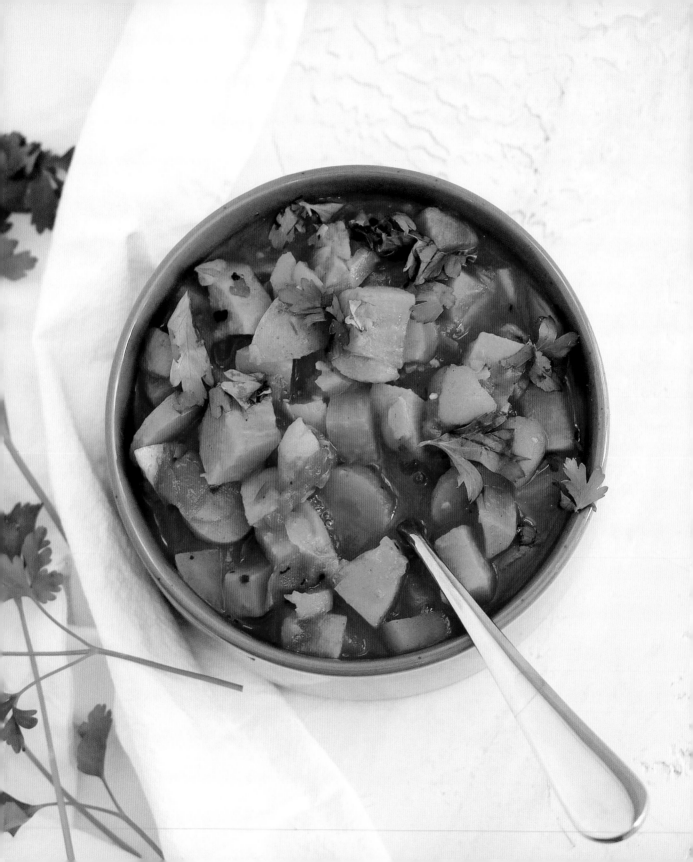

SWEET & SAVORY MOROCCAN VEGETABLE TAGINE

Sometimes stew sounds like the perfect meal, but maybe the timing isn't so perfect on a busy weeknight. Enter this bright and flavorful tagine, which comes together in minutes instead of hours, while no flavor is spared. Use a heavy-bottomed pot with a tight-fitting lid, like a Dutch oven, to get fast and delicious results, and get ready for your taste buds to go on vacation!

YIELD: 8 CUPS (1.9 L)
PREP TIME: 10 MINUTES
COOKING TIME: 20 MINUTES

2 tbsp (30 ml) olive oil

1 medium yellow onion, finely chopped

1 tbsp (7 g) minced garlic

2 large carrots, sliced thin

4 small to medium Yukon gold potatoes, cubed into ½-inch (1.3-cm) pieces

2 small sweet potatoes, peeled and cubed into ½-inch (1.3-cm) pieces

2 tbsp (30 g) harissa paste

1 tsp salt

1 tsp ground coriander

1 tsp cinnamon

½ tsp ground turmeric

1 (32-oz [907-g]) container vegetable broth

1 (14.5-oz [411-g]) jar petite fire-roasted diced tomatoes

½ cup (73 g) chopped dried apricots

Juice of 1 lemon

¼ cup (15 g) fresh parsley, finely chopped

Heat the olive oil in a large heavy pot or Dutch oven over medium-high heat. Add the onion, garlic, carrots, potatoes and sweet potatoes and sauté for 5 minutes. Add the harissa, salt, coriander, cinnamon and turmeric and stir to combine. Stir in the vegetable broth, diced tomatoes and dried apricots. Bring to a low boil, cover with a tight-fitting lid and cook for 15 minutes, or until the vegetables are soft.

Stir in the lemon juice and top with fresh parsley before serving.

QUICK TIP: I find frozen cubed sweet potatoes with no other ingredients added (often fire-roasted for even more flavor) in the freezer section of our grocery store. They're a great way to speed up prep, and don't take much longer to cook—especially in a stew-type dish like this!

ROASTED GREEK VEGGIE BOWLS WITH ZUCCHINI HUMMUS

These veggie-packed bowls are full of roasted vegetable goodness that will take you straight to the Mediterranean. But let's be honest, the hummus is what makes these bowls insanely good! It's the easiest thing to make, pairs well with so many dishes and takes a simple meal to the next level. I can't wait for you to try it and serve it with everything!

YIELD: 4 BOWLS
PREP TIME: 7 MINUTES
COOKING TIME: 20 MINUTES

FOR THE ROASTED VEGETABLES

1 red bell pepper, cubed

1 green bell pepper, cubed

1 medium eggplant, cubed

1 red onion, sliced thin

1 large zucchini, halved lengthwise then sliced into ¼-inch (6-mm)-thick pieces

2 cups (298 g) grape tomatoes

2 tbsp (17 g) minced garlic

2 tbsp (30 ml) olive oil

1 tsp salt

½ tsp black pepper

FOR THE HUMMUS

1 cup (124 g) peeled and diced zucchini

⅓ cup (80 ml) tahini

2 tbsp (30 ml) lemon juice

2 cloves garlic, minced

2 tsp (2 g) cumin

½ tsp salt

FOR SERVING

4 cups spring mix

Chopped fresh dill, cilantro and parsley, for garnish

For the roasted vegetables: Preheat the oven to 425°F (218°C). Line a baking sheet with parchment paper. Arrange the bell peppers, eggplant, onion, zucchini, tomatoes and garlic in a single layer, using two sheet pans if needed. Drizzle with the olive oil and season with salt and pepper. Transfer to the oven and bake for 20 minutes, or until the vegetables are tender.

For the hummus: Add the zucchini, tahini, lemon juice, garlic, cumin and salt to a high-speed blender or mini food processor. Blend until smooth and creamy. Transfer to the refrigerator until ready to serve.

To serve: Serve the roasted vegetables in bowls over 1 cup of spring mix, topped with a scoop of hummus and fresh herbs to garnish.

QUICK TIP: Keep this hummus on hand in the fridge, at all times. It's a dip, it's a dressing, it goes on everything. I especially love making this hummus in the summertime when garden zucchini is abundant and we're searching for new ways to use it up!

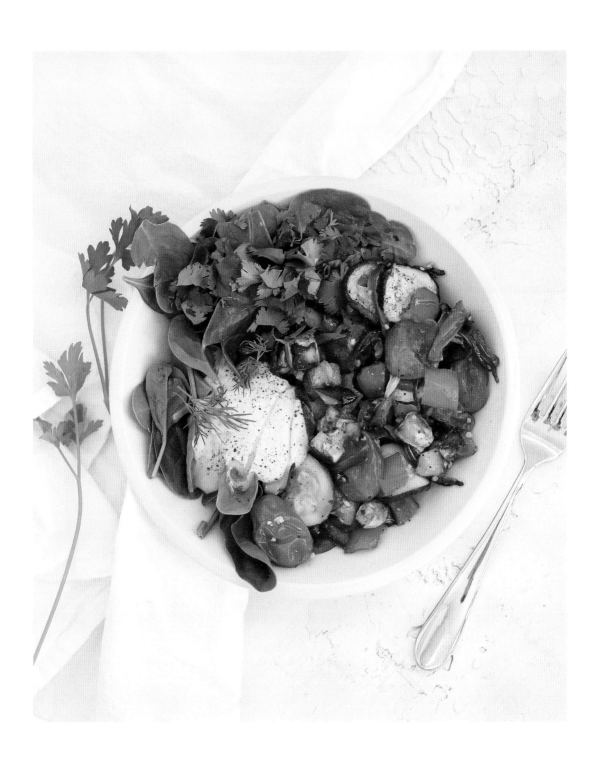

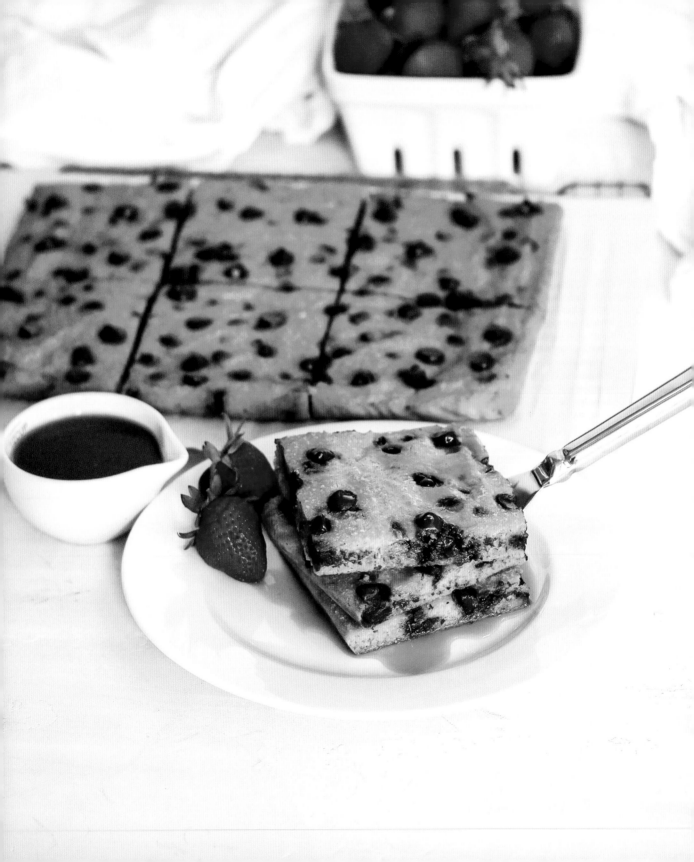

BRUNCH IN A HURRY

Brunch: for when it's too late for breakfast, but a little early for lunch. When you're entertaining and want to cook breakfast, but don't want everyone to get there too early. It's honestly my favorite meal of the day, and a great excuse to make something a little extra special! If you're ready for brunch, I've got you more than covered in this chapter with sheet pan pancakes, baked "n'oatmeal," savory sausage waffles, shakshuka, tacos, egg-free dishes and beyond.

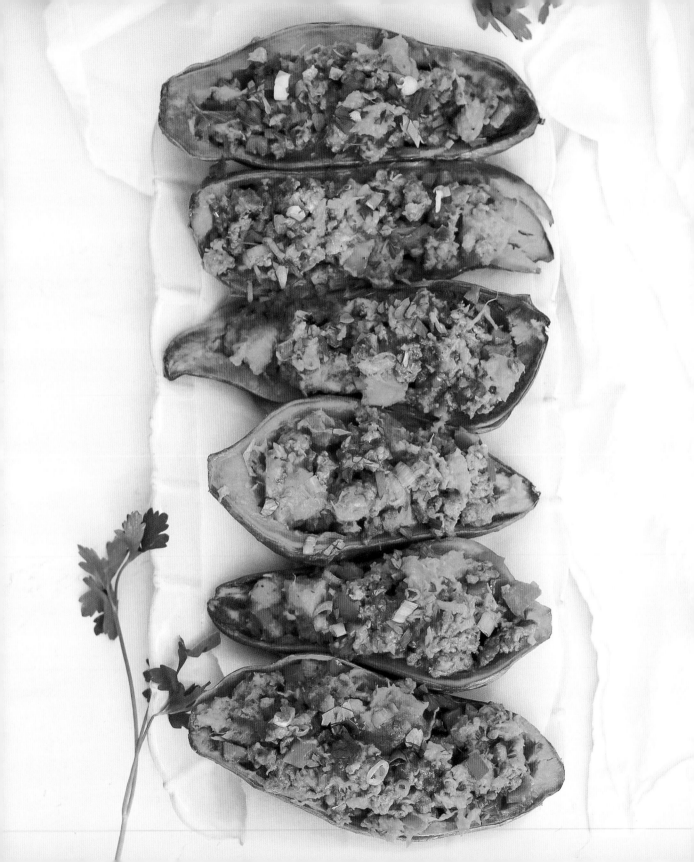

SAUSAGE-STUFFED SWEET POTATO HALVES

"Egg-free breakfasts" are a common request I receive, and this savory breakfast fits the bill, whether you are an egg lover or not. Sausage and sweet potato is a match made in heaven, and this mixture uses just the right amount of veggies to add some color and flavor. This one is great for entertaining, but also makes a perfect "make-ahead" breakfast to reheat throughout the week!

YIELD: 6 SWEET POTATO HALVES
PREP TIME: 7 MINUTES
COOKING TIME: 18 MINUTES

3 small to medium sweet potatoes

1 lb (454 g) ground pork breakfast sausage

1 small red bell pepper, diced

½ medium yellow onion, finely diced

¼ cup (12 g) sliced scallion, plus more for garnish

2 cloves garlic, minced

½ tsp garlic powder

½ tsp onion powder

½ tsp salt

½ tsp black pepper

Finely chopped fresh parsley and hot sauce, for garnish

Rinse the sweet potatoes, then use a fork or the tip of a sharp knife to poke a few small holes in each one. Wrap each potato in a damp paper towel, then place them all in the microwave. Cook for 3 minutes per side, or until soft.

Heat a large skillet over medium to medium-high heat and add the sausage. Cook for 7 minutes, or until crumbled and browned. Stir in the bell pepper, onion, scallion, garlic, garlic powder, onion powder, salt and pepper and continue to cook for 4 to 5 minutes, or until the vegetables are tender.

Slice the sweet potatoes in half lengthwise and scoop out the flesh (leaving enough behind to keep the skins intact), adding it to the cooked sausage mixture. Stir the mixture together to combine, then spoon back into the sweet potato skins.

Serve hot with additional scallions, fresh parsley and hot sauce to garnish.

QUICK TIP: Not a fan of the microwave? Bake the sweet potatoes in the oven ahead of time, and keep them on hand in the fridge for a quick meal.

LOADED-UP COWBOY STEAK & POTATO HASH

This one's for my meaty breakfast lovers who appreciate a warm, hearty skillet with a southwestern flair. Think "seasoned home fries," but add steak and finish with fresh herbs, sliced jalapeño and a good drizzle of ranch dressing. Is your mouth watering yet? Let's get cookin'!

YIELD: 4 SERVINGS
PREP TIME: 7 MINUTES
COOKING TIME: 17 MINUTES

1 tbsp (15 g) ghee

1 rib eye steak, cut into 1-inch (2.5-cm) bite-sized pieces

12 small Yukon gold potatoes, quartered

1 medium red bell pepper, diced

½ medium yellow onion, diced

2 tsp (4 g) minced garlic

½ tsp salt

½ tsp black pepper

½ tsp chili powder

½ tsp oregano

Fresh chopped parsley, thinly sliced jalapeño and Paleo-friendly ranch dressing, for garnish

Melt the ghee in a skillet over medium-high heat. Add the steak pieces and cook until browned on all sides, 4 to 5 minutes. Transfer to a plate and set aside.

Reduce the heat to medium and add the potatoes, bell pepper, onion, garlic, salt, pepper, chili powder and oregano to the skillet. Cook until the potatoes are fork-tender, 8 to 10 minutes.

Stir the steak back in and cook for 1 to 2 more minutes, or until warm. Garnish with parsley, jalapeño and a drizzle of ranch.

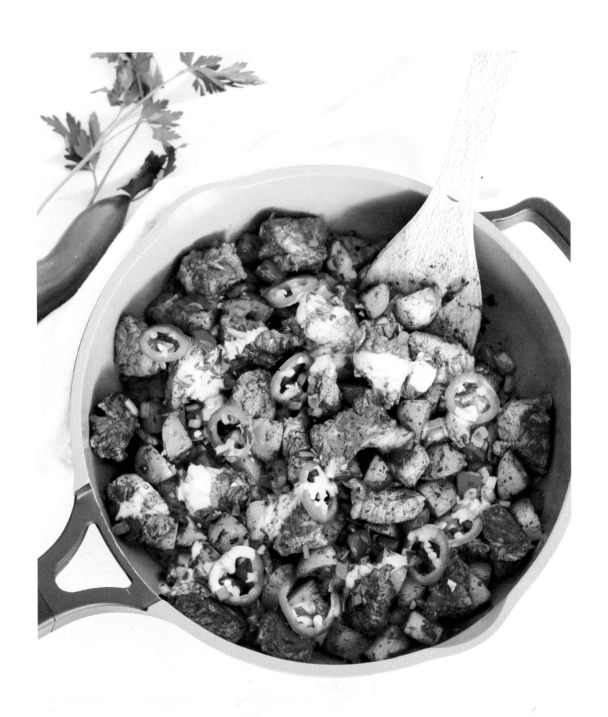

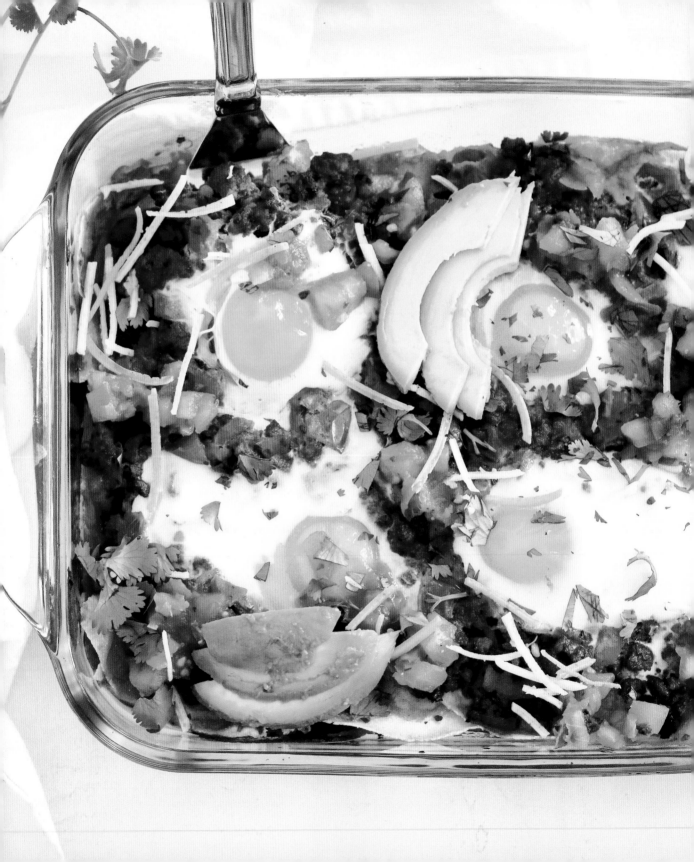

SOUTHWEST HUEVOS RANCHEROS CASSEROLE

Sweet potato and chorizo is another dream team for me. There's just something about the combination of savory and sweet-and-spicy that works so perfectly together. In this dish, it's layered up with tortillas in between and all of the fixings on top for a delicious play on huevos rancheros, done casserole style.

YIELD: 6 SERVINGS
PREP TIME: 10 MINUTES
COOKING TIME: 20 MINUTES

Avocado oil spray

1 lb (454 g) ground chorizo sausage

1 (14-oz [396-g]) can petite fire-roasted diced tomatoes

1 (15-oz [425-g]) can sweet potato puree

1 tsp salt

½ tsp chili powder

½ tsp garlic powder

¼ tsp cumin

⅛ tsp cayenne pepper

8 Paleo-friendly tortillas

6 eggs

½ avocado, thinly sliced, for garnish

½ cup (120 ml) pico de gallo, for garnish

¼ cup (4 g) cilantro, roughly chopped, for garnish

¼ cup (12 g) scallions, thinly sliced, for garnish

1 jalapeño pepper, thinly sliced, for garnish

¼ cup (28 g) dairy-free shredded cheese, for garnish (optional)

Preheat the oven to 400°F (204°C). Spray a 9 x 13–inch (23 x 33–cm) baking dish with avocado oil spray and set aside.

Heat a medium skillet over medium-high heat and add the chorizo. Cook until crumbled and browned, about 8 minutes, then stir in the diced tomatoes and turn off the heat.

In a medium bowl, stir the sweet potato puree, salt, chili powder, garlic powder, cumin and cayenne until smooth.

Tear the tortillas into about four to five pieces each, so they're easy to layer in the bottom of the baking dish. Arrange them so that they roughly cover the bottom, then add half of the sweet potato mixture and spread it evenly over the tortillas. Add half of the chorizo mixture and spread it evenly over the sweet potato mixture. Repeat with one more layer of tortillas, sweet potato mixture and chorizo mixture. Make six wells in the top of the chorizo mixture and crack an egg into each.

Transfer to the oven and bake for 10 to 12 minutes, or until the egg whites are set and the yolks are still runny.

Top with avocado, pico de gallo, cilantro, scallions, jalapeño and dairy-free cheese (if using) to garnish and serve hot.

CRISPY SALMON CAKES WITH LEMON AIOLI & GREENS

To me, these salmon cakes define brunch, with crispy, savory lunch vibes, but topped with a fresh lemon aioli and served over spring mix to lighten them up. These are great in the morning with some fresh berries and a latte, but can also mix up your workweek lunches when served chilled over greens as an easy salad to grab and go.

YIELD: 8 SALMON CAKES
PREP TIME: 10 MINUTES
COOKING TIME: 10 MINUTES

FOR THE LEMON AIOLI

⅓ cup (80 ml) avocado oil
2 tbsp (30 ml) coconut milk
1 egg
1 tsp minced garlic
½ tsp salt
½ tsp black pepper
¼ tsp Dijon mustard
Zest of 1 lemon
Juice of ½ lemon

FOR THE SALMON CAKES

2 (6-oz [170-g]) cans salmon, drained
2 eggs
1 tbsp (15 ml) Dijon mustard
2 tsp (5 g) onion powder
1 tsp minced garlic
½ tsp salt, plus more to taste
½ tsp black pepper
½ tsp smoked paprika
¼ cup (33 g) tapioca flour
3 tbsp (45 ml) avocado oil

FOR SERVING

Mixed greens
Lemon wedges

To make the lemon aioli: In a blender, combine the oil, coconut milk and egg. Pulse until evenly combined. Add the garlic, salt, pepper, Dijon, lemon zest and lemon juice and continue to blend until combined and thickened to a mayo-like texture or slightly thinner. Transfer to a small bowl and refrigerate until ready to serve.

To make the salmon cakes: In a medium bowl, combine the salmon, eggs, Dijon, onion powder, minced garlic, salt, pepper, paprika and tapioca flour and mix with a fork. In a large skillet over medium-high heat, heat the avocado oil. Use a ¼-cup (60-ml) measuring cup to scoop the mixture into your hands and form into round patties ½ to 1 inch (1.3 to 2.5 cm) thick. Place in the hot pan and cook for 5 minutes on each side, or until golden brown. Season with additional salt, if you like.

To serve: Serve the hot salmon cakes over mixed greens, topped with the lemon aioli and a squeeze of fresh lemon juice. They also taste great chilled the next day!

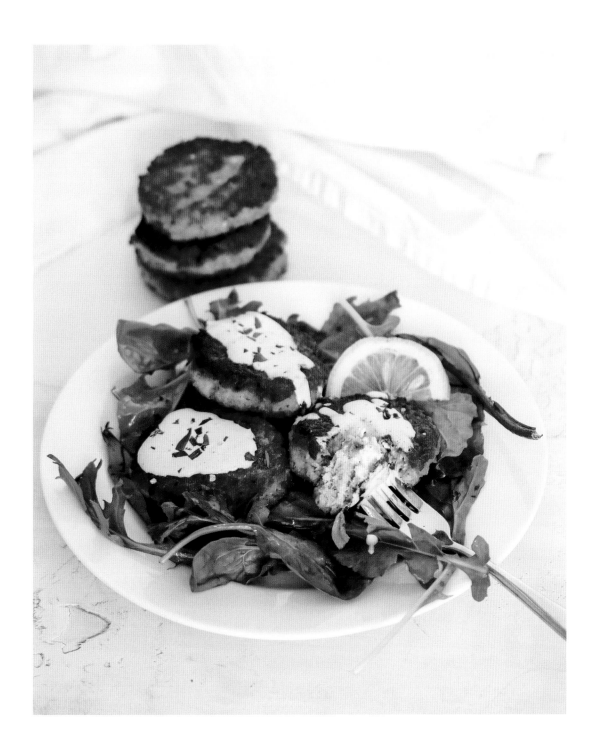

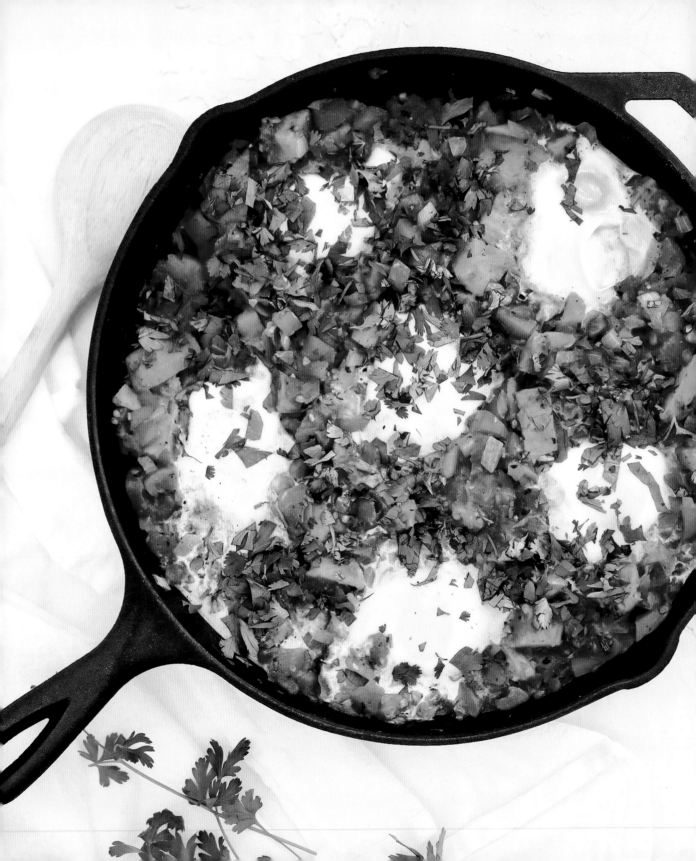

SHORTCUT STOVETOP SHAKSHUKA

My take on the classic shakshuka skillet breakfast involves bulking it up a bit with fire-roasted sweet potatoes. They add so much great flavor and texture, while still allowing those classic smoky spices to shine through. Serve this up hot with lots of fresh herbs and enjoy!

YIELD: 6 SERVINGS
PREP TIME: 5 MINUTES
COOKING TIME: 21 MINUTES

2 tsp (10 ml) olive oil

1 medium yellow onion, diced

1 red bell pepper, diced

2 tsp (4 g) minced garlic

2 tsp (4 g) paprika

1 tsp cumin

¼ tsp chipotle powder

1 (16-oz [453-g]) bag fire-roasted sweet potatoes, cubed

2 (14.5-oz [411-g]) cans petite fire-roasted diced tomatoes

½ tsp salt

½ tsp black pepper

6 large eggs

¼ cup (4 g) fresh cilantro, chopped, for garnish

¼ cup (6 g) fresh parsley, chopped, for garnish

In a large skillet over medium heat, heat the olive oil. Add the onion and bell pepper and cook for 5 minutes. Stir in the garlic, paprika, cumin and chipotle powder and cook for 1 more minute. Add the frozen sweet potatoes and diced tomatoes and bring to a simmer. Simmer for 5 to 7 minutes, or until the sweet potatoes are warm and fork-tender. Season with salt and pepper and stir.

Use a wooden spoon to make six small wells in the sauce and crack an egg into each well. Cover the pan and cook for 5 to 8 minutes, or until the eggs are done to your liking (I like a set white and a runny yolk).

Garnish with the fresh herbs and serve hot.

QUICK TIP: I use a bag of frozen, fully cooked fire-roasted sweet potatoes in this recipe. They come pre-cubed, which is such a time saver! If you can't find these, you can use raw sweet potato and cube it yourself. You may need to increase the cook time by around 5 minutes to get them nice and tender.

HASH BROWN & SAUSAGE WAFFLES

A full breakfast walks into a waffle iron and becomes . . . a crispy, savory waffle! Pork sausage, egg, hash browns, maple syrup, dried herbs and a little "cheesy" flair, all in one golden-brown vessel ready to be topped as you wish. If I could eat one breakfast for the rest of forever, these waffles would be it!

YIELD: 4 WAFFLES
PREP TIME: 5 MINUTES
COOKING TIME: 15 MINUTES

4 oz (113 g) ground pork breakfast sausage

1 egg

¼ cup (20 g) nutritional yeast

4 oz (113 g) refrigerated hash browns

1 tbsp (15 ml) maple syrup

1 tbsp (15 ml) coconut milk

½ tsp garlic powder

½ tsp dried chives

¼ tsp sage

¼ tsp thyme

¼ tsp salt

¼ tsp black pepper

Avocado oil spray

Mixed greens, fried egg and hot sauce, for topping (optional)

In a mixing bowl, combine the sausage, egg, nutritional yeast, hash browns, maple syrup, coconut milk, garlic powder, chives, sage, thyme, salt and pepper and stir until well combined.

Spray a waffle iron heated to medium with avocado oil spray. Add the waffle mixture to fill, and cook for 15 minutes, or until golden-brown and crispy.

Eat alone or serve in stacks over mixed greens, topped with a crispy fried egg and a drizzle of hot sauce.

QUICK TIP: If you've got a little more time to spend, and the waffle iron is already heated—go ahead and double (or even triple) this recipe and save the rest for easy breakfasts any time. You can store leftover waffles in the fridge, or even the freezer, then reheat them in the microwave or air fryer when you're ready to enjoy.

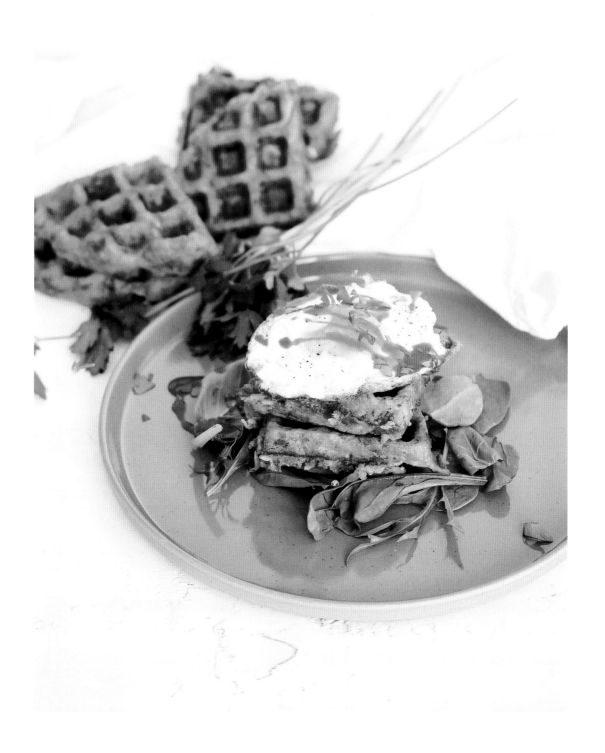

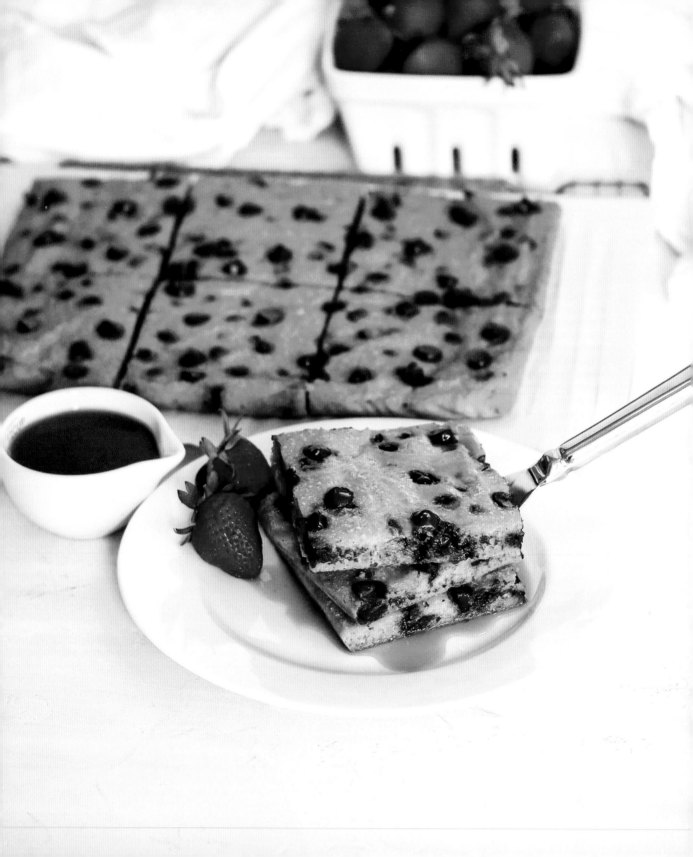

CHOCOLATE CHIP SHEET PAN PANCAKES

Why pour and flip and stack twelve times over when you can pour and bake and you're done? Sheet pan pancakes are my Sunday morning best friend. I'm not the world's best flipper, and these turn out so much fluffier and are literally foolproof. The chocolate chips? They're just the icing on the (pan)cake.

YIELD: 12 SERVINGS
PREP TIME: 10 MINUTES
COOKING TIME: 15 TO 20 MINUTES

1⅓ cups (166 g) coconut flour

1⅓ cups (150 g) tapioca flour

2 tsp (9 g) baking powder

1 tsp baking soda

½ tsp salt

2 cups (480 ml) dairy-free milk

6 eggs

¼ cup (60 ml) melted grass-fed butter or coconut oil, melted then cooled

¼ cup (60 ml) honey

2 tsp (10 ml) vanilla

1½ cups (252 g) dairy-free chocolate chips, divided

Maple syrup, for topping

Preheat the oven to 400°F (204°C). Line a rimmed baking sheet with parchment paper and set aside.

Add the coconut flour, tapioca flour, baking powder, baking soda and salt to a large bowl and stir to combine. Add the milk, eggs, cooled melted butter, honey and vanilla and stir until well mixed. Stir in 1 cup (168 g) of chocolate chips. Use a rubber spatula to pour the pancake batter onto the lined baking sheet. Sprinkle the remaining ½ cup (84 g) of chocolate chips over top.

Transfer to the oven and bake for 15 to 20 minutes, or until light golden on top and set in the middle.

Slice into squares and serve warm, topped with warm maple syrup.

PUMPKIN SPICE BAKED N'OATMEAL BITES

Soft and fluffy baked oatmeal texture, warm pumpkin spice flavor, sweet coconut sugar and nutty pecans. These muffins are fall in a bite but honestly, they're just perfect to be eaten year-round. Serve them warm, broken up with a little milk and a spoon or eat them straight-up, muffin style. Either way, the whole family will love them!

YIELD: 12 MUFFIN BITES
PREP TIME: 7 MINUTES
COOKING TIME: 23 MINUTES

1½ cups (140 g) unsweetened shredded coconut

¾ cup (82 g) chopped pecans, plus extra for topping

½ cup (100 g) coconut sugar, plus extra for topping

2 tbsp (16 g) coconut flour

1½ tsp (4 g) cinnamon

½ tsp nutmeg

¼ tsp ground ginger

¼ tsp ground clove

1 tsp baking soda

½ tsp salt

4 eggs, whisked

1 cup (240 ml) dairy-free milk

1 cup (245 g) pumpkin puree

1 tbsp (15 ml) vanilla

Preheat the oven to 350°F (176°C). Line a 12-cup muffin tin with parchment paper cups and set aside.

To a large bowl, add all of the ingredients and stir until well combined. Distribute equally among the twelve cups and top with a little extra chopped pecans and coconut sugar. Transfer to the oven and bake for 20 to 23 minutes, or until the bites are set.

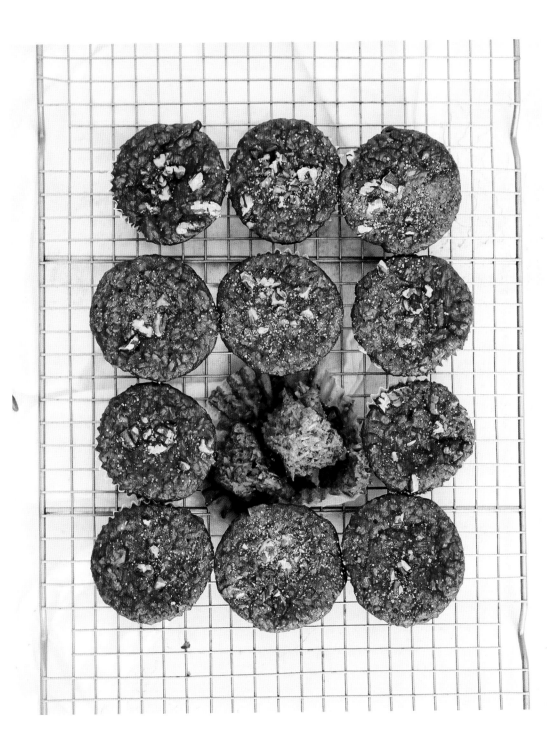

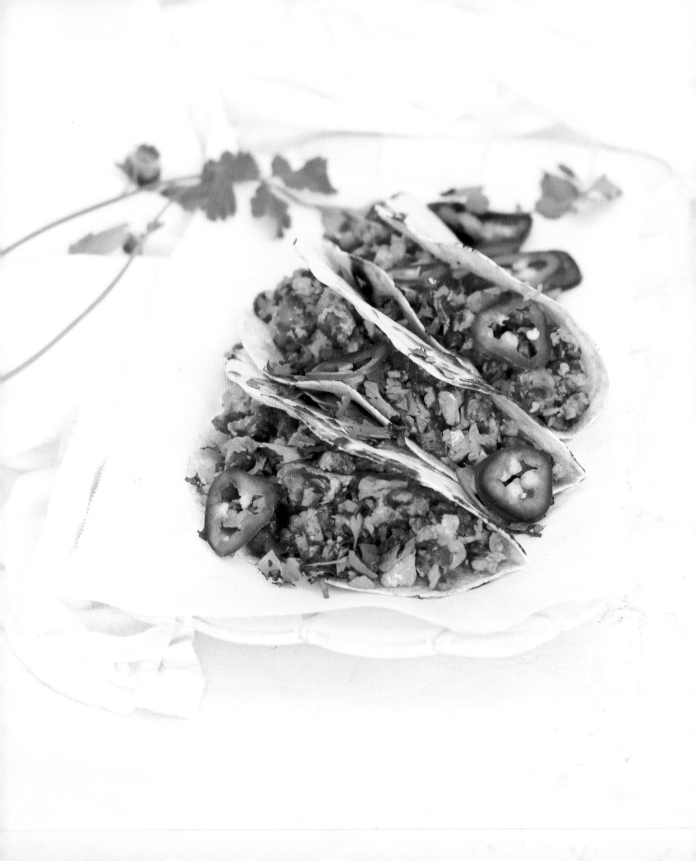

CHORIZO & EGG BREAKFAST TACOS

Chorizo sausage is a nostalgic food for me from my childhood, one I discovered through many nights sleeping over at my best friend's house growing up. Her mom would often make chorizo and eggs for us in the morning, and it was a whole new thing for me—flavors I had never experienced before. I loved it so much, I had to make it myself at home! Luckily, it's super simple to do—hard to mess up, really! Serve the mixture in charred tortillas and you'll have a breakfast that tastes like Mexican comfort food with super minimal effort.

YIELD: 6 TACOS
PREP TIME: 2 MINUTES
COOKING TIME: 17 MINUTES

1 lb (454 g) ground chorizo

6 eggs, whisked

6 Paleo-friendly tortillas

¼ cup (4 g) fresh cilantro, chopped

1 small jalapeño pepper, sliced thin

Hot sauce (optional)

Heat a nonstick skillet over medium and put the chorizo in it. Cook until crumbled and browned, about 8 minutes. Use a wooden spoon to break the chorizo into very small pieces. Reduce the heat to low and move the chorizo to the sides of the pan, creating a well in the center. Add the whisked eggs to the center and continue to cook, moving the eggs around and breaking them into pieces for 3 to 4 minutes, or until the eggs are just set.

Char the tortillas over a low flame on a gas stovetop (or, if using an electric stovetop, warm in a pan over medium heat).

Fill the tortillas with the chorizo and egg mixture and top with cilantro, jalapeño and hot sauce (if using).

PROSCIUTTO & SPINACH EGG CUPS

My favorite part about these easy egg cups? Just how crispy that prosciutto gets in less than 15 minutes. It's honestly incredible. I love the salty bite of the meat, the perfectly slightly runny yolk (you can cook it fully if you like!), and the garlicky spinach surprise hidden between the layers. Make these to serve for the family or try them for meal prep! They reheat beautifully.

YIELD: 12 CUPS
PREP TIME: 5 MINUTES
COOKING TIME: 18 MINUTES

Avocado oil spray

12 slices prosciutto

1 tsp olive oil

3 cups (90 g) loosely packed baby spinach

2 tsp (4 g) minced garlic

12 eggs

Salt and black pepper, for seasoning

Finely chopped fresh parsley and red pepper flakes, for garnish

Preheat the oven to 425°F (218°C). Spray each well of a 12-cup muffin tin with avocado oil spray. Line the bottom and sides of each muffin cup with 1 slice of prosciutto, using small pieces to cover any holes as needed.

Heat the olive oil in a skillet over medium heat. Add the spinach and garlic and sauté for 2 to 3 minutes, or until just wilted. Use a spoon to add 1 to 2 tablespoons (2 to 4 g) of the spinach mixture to each cup of the muffin tin.

Crack 1 egg into each muffin cup. Season each cup with a small amount of salt and pepper, then transfer to the oven and bake for 10 to 15 minutes, depending on how cooked you like your yolk.

Garnish with parsley and red pepper flakes, and serve hot. Store leftovers in the fridge and reheat as needed.

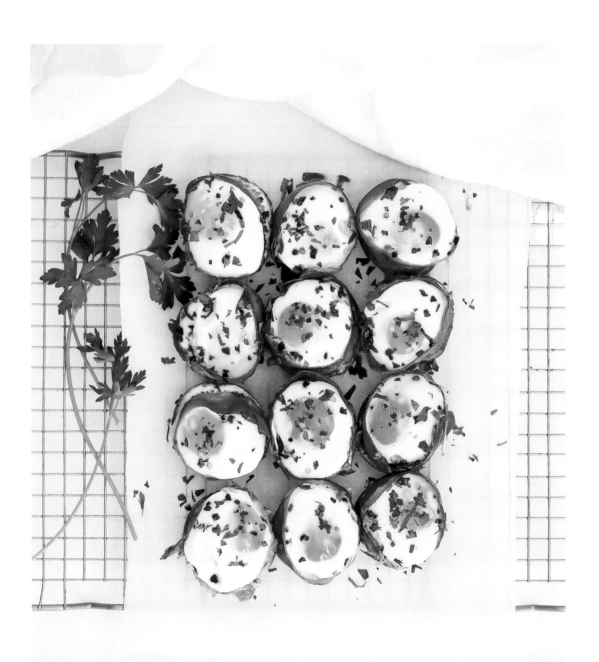

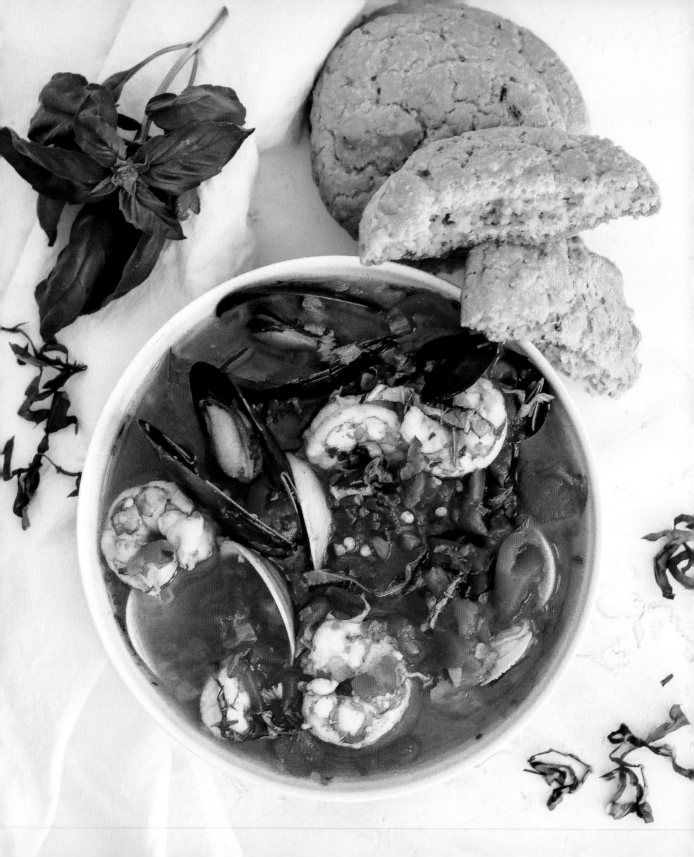

SPEEDY SOUPS & SALADS

You may read "soups and salads" and think, "Oh, those are some add-ons or side dishes" . . . nope. These are real-deal, full-on meals, and some of my very favorite recipes await you in this chapter! Italian, Southern, classic American, Thai, Jamaican, Greek: we're traveling all around the world with these quick and filling recipes you'll come back to again and again!

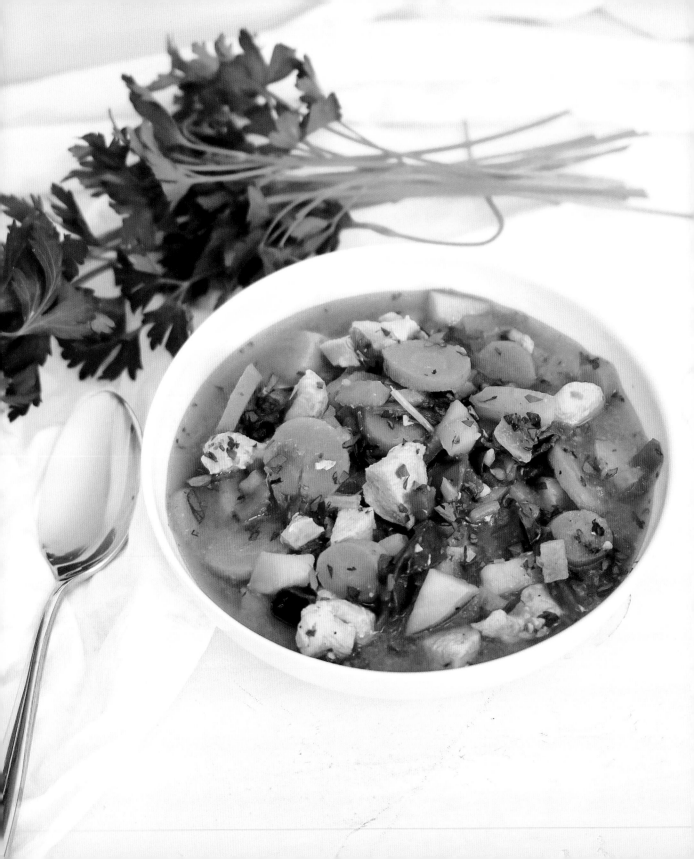

CHUNKY CHICKEN & ROASTED VEGETABLE SOUP

This is the chunky chicken and veggie soup from a can that I worshipped in my childhood (and beyond), but done grown-up style with fresh vegetables, big chunks of juicy chicken, savory dried herbs and spices and some roasted tomatoes to add depth and extra deliciousness. This is one soup our whole family can't get enough of, and I love how nutrient dense it is for something that just tastes so good.

YIELD: 10 CUPS (2.4 L)
PREP TIME: 7 MINUTES
COOKING TIME: 22 MINUTES

1 tbsp (15 ml) olive oil

2 chicken breasts, cut into ½- to 1-inch (1.3- to 2.5-cm) bite-sized pieces

4 medium Yukon gold potatoes, cut into ¼-inch (6-mm) pieces

2 large carrots, sliced thin

2 celery stalks, halved lengthwise then thinly sliced

½ medium yellow onion, diced

1 (14.5-oz [411-g]) can petite fire-roasted diced tomatoes

½ tsp onion powder

½ tsp garlic powder

½ tsp chili powder

½ tsp oregano

½ tsp dried chives

½ tsp salt, plus more to taste

½ tsp black pepper, plus more to taste

1 (32-oz [907-g]) container chicken bone broth

1 cup (30 g) chopped baby spinach

¼ cup (15 g) chopped parsley

In a large pot or Dutch oven over medium-high heat, heat the olive oil. Add the chicken, potatoes, carrots, celery and onion and sauté for 5 minutes. Stir in the diced tomatoes, onion powder, garlic powder, chili powder, oregano, dried chives, salt, pepper and bone broth and bring to a low boil. Cover with a tight-fitting lid and cook for 10 to 15 minutes, or until the vegetables are tender and chicken is fully opaque and cooked through. In a Dutch oven, this will take closer to 10 minutes, whereas a traditional pot will be more like 15.

Stir in the baby spinach and chopped parsley, and cook for 2 more minutes, or until the greens are just wilted.

Serve hot, with additional salt and pepper to taste.

SMOKY SHRIMP & SWEET POTATO CHOWDER

The first time my husband visited me when we were dating long distance, we cooked this recipe together! Well, mostly I cooked, and he washed the dishes. These days I cook, and I also wash the dishes. But he does a million other things, and I love him even more now than I did then. Back to the soup: It's smoky, it's sweet, it's so many flavors all in one that I can hardly describe it—and there's bacon on top. It's unforgettable, and I can't wait for you to try it!

YIELD: 8 CUPS (1.9 L)
PREP TIME: 7 MINUTES
COOKING TIME: 16 MINUTES

1 tbsp (15 ml) avocado oil

3 medium sweet potatoes, peeled and cut into ½-inch (1.3-cm) cubes

½ medium yellow onion, diced

½ tsp minced garlic

½ tsp minced ginger

2 cups (480 ml) coconut milk

2 cups (480 ml) chicken broth

1 cup (30 g) baby spinach

1 lb (454 g) shrimp, peeled and deveined

½ tsp dried Italian herb seasoning

½ tsp salt

½ tsp black pepper

¼ tsp red pepper flakes

¼ tsp nutmeg

Fresh chopped parsley and fully cooked bacon, for garnish

In a large pot or Dutch oven over medium-high to high heat, heat the avocado oil. Add the sweet potatoes, onion, garlic, ginger, coconut milk and chicken broth and bring to a boil. Cover and cook for 10 minutes, or until the sweet potatoes are soft.

Reduce the heat to a simmer and use an immersion blender to blend the soup until "half-blended," or smooth with some chunks of vegetables remaining. Add the spinach, shrimp, Italian herb seasoning, salt, pepper, red pepper flakes and nutmeg and stir to combine. Simmer until the shrimp is opaque and the spinach is wilted, 3 to 4 minutes.

Serve hot and garnished with chopped parsley and crumbled bacon.

QUICK TIP: Crispy oven bacon is my thing, and I always make enough to have extra waiting in the fridge for dishes just like this. Adding bacon to the top honestly makes the dish!

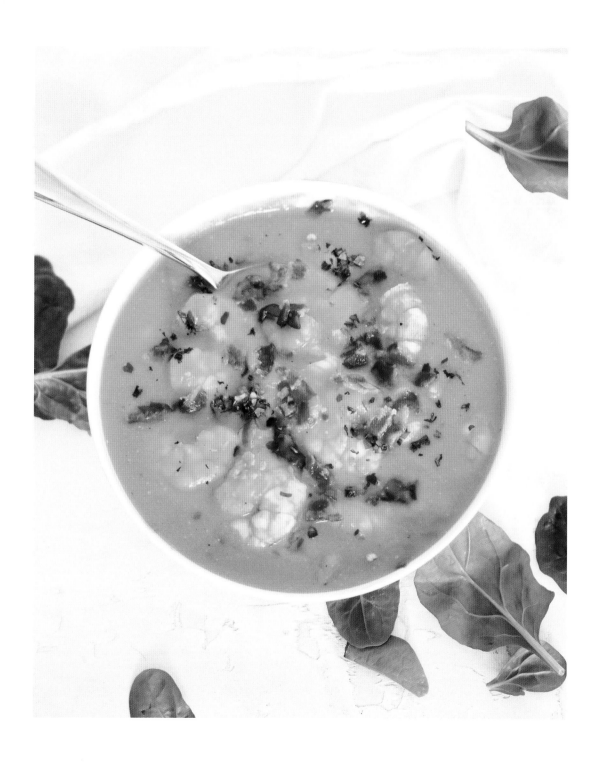

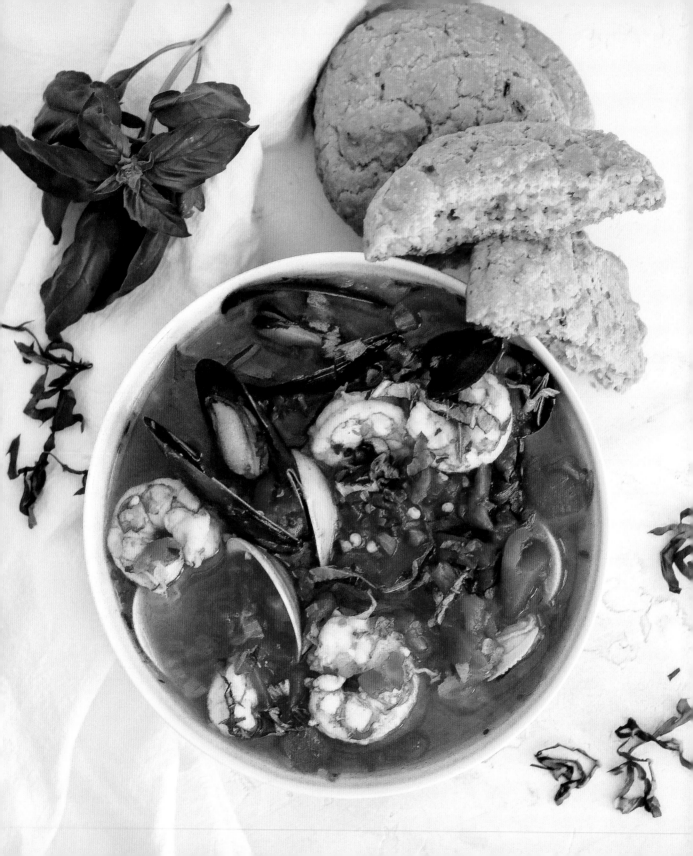

SEAFOOD CIOPPINO WITH GARLIC-HERB BISCUITS

Need a dish to impress? This beautiful Italian seafood stew is it. Cioppino is a "fisherman's stew" with Italian herbs, fresh seafood and a tomato base. One thing it's almost never: done in under 30 minutes. Defy all odds with this simplified version, and then blow them away with a crisp, golden garlic biscuit baked in no time flat. Ready, set, go!

YIELD: 8 SERVINGS
PREP TIME: 10 MINUTES
COOKING TIME: 15 MINUTES

FOR THE BISCUITS

2 cups (250 g) almond flour

⅓ cup (75 g) grass-fed butter or ghee, melted

2 tsp (9 g) baking powder

1 tsp garlic powder

½ tsp dried Italian herb seasoning

½ tsp salt

2 eggs

Flakey sea salt, for topping

FOR THE CIOPPINO

1 tbsp (15 ml) olive oil

½ cup (80 g) shallot, finely chopped

1 tbsp (8 g) minced garlic

2 (14.5-oz [411-g]) cans petite diced tomatoes

2 cups (480 ml) chicken broth

2 cups (480 ml) dry white wine, or additional chicken broth

2 tsp (11 g) dried Italian herb seasoning

1 tsp paprika

½ tsp garlic powder

¼ tsp red pepper flakes

1 lb (454 g) shrimp, peeled and deveined

1 lb (454 g) whole clams, fully cooked

1 lb (454 g) mussels, fully cooked

½ cup (12 g) loosely packed fresh basil leaves, roughly chopped

½ tsp salt, plus more to taste

½ tsp black pepper, plus more to taste

Fresh chopped parsley, for garnish

To make the biscuits: Preheat the oven to 350°F (176°C). Line a baking sheet with parchment paper and set aside. In a medium bowl, combine the almond flour, butter, baking powder, garlic powder, Italian herb seasoning, salt and eggs until mixed. Use a cookie dough scoop or measuring spoon to scoop out 2 tablespoons (30 g) of dough. Shape into round biscuits and slightly flatten the top. Arrange on the lined baking sheet and sprinkle the tops with sea salt. Transfer to the oven and bake for 15 minutes, or until light golden brown.

To make the cioppino: While the biscuits cook, make the stew. In a large pot or Dutch oven over medium to medium-high heat, heat the olive oil. Add the shallot and garlic and cook until softened and fragrant, about 2 minutes. Add the tomatoes, broth, wine (if using), Italian herb seasoning, paprika, garlic powder and red pepper flakes and bring to a low boil. Stir in the shrimp, clams and mussels and reduce the heat to a simmer. Cook for 8 to 10 minutes, or until the shrimp is opaque and the clams and mussels open. Discard any shellfish that do not open.

Stir in the fresh basil and season with additional salt and pepper to taste. Garnish with fresh parsley and serve hot with the warm biscuits.

LOADED CAULIFLOWER SOUP WITH BACON & JALAPEÑO

This soup combines the feel-good cauliflower with the tastes-good potato and creates the most deliciously rich and creamy soup. When topped with bacon, jalapeño and scallion, it's a veggie-packed soup you'll *crave*.

YIELD: 8 CUPS (1.9 L)
PREP TIME: 5 MINUTES
COOKING TIME: 18 MINUTES

2 tbsp (30 g) ghee

2 cups (300 g) diced gold potatoes

2 tsp (8 g) minced garlic

1 (16-oz [453-g]) bag cauliflower rice

1 (32-oz [907-g]) container chicken broth

2 cups (480 ml) dairy-free milk

1 cup (146 g) raw cashews

¼ cup (20 g) nutritional yeast

1 tsp onion powder

1 tsp garlic powder

1 tsp salt, plus more to taste

1 tsp black pepper, plus more to taste

8 slices fully cooked bacon, for garnish

½ jalapeño, seeded and thinly sliced, for garnish

⅓ cup (16 g) thinly sliced scallion, for garnish

In a large pot over medium to medium-high heat, heat the ghee. Add the potatoes and garlic and sauté for 3 minutes. Stir in the cauliflower rice and cook for another 3 minutes. Add the chicken broth and bring to a low boil. Cover and cook until the potatoes are tender, about 10 minutes.

In a blender, combine the milk, cashews, nutritional yeast, onion powder, garlic powder, salt and pepper. Blend for about 1 minute, or until smooth and creamy, then pour into the cooked soup and stir to combine. Heat for an additional 2 minutes to warm through.

Season the soup with additional salt and pepper to taste, then garnish with the bacon, jalapeño and scallion.

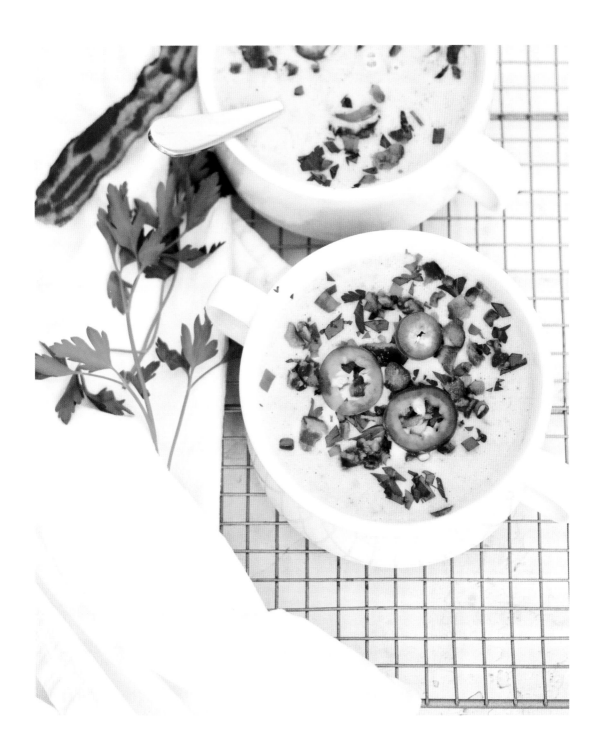

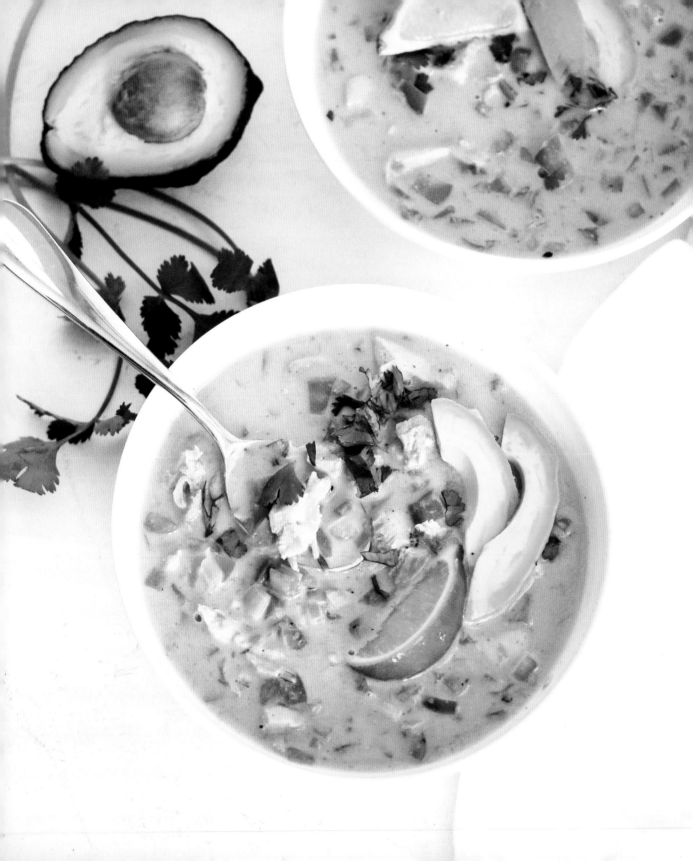

CREAMY GREEN CHILE CHICKEN SOUP

Mild yet flavorful, this soup packs a zesty punch without overwhelming you with heat. Flavors don't have to take forever to develop—this one is so fast! It's made creamy with a "cashew cream" that whips up super quick in the blender while the soup cooks. Mix it all together, and don't skimp on the garnishes!

YIELD: 8 CUPS (1.9 L)
PREP TIME: 5 MINUTES
COOKING TIME: 25 MINUTES

2 tsp (10 ml) avocado oil

1 medium white or yellow onion, diced

1 green bell pepper, finely diced

2 medium carrots, finely diced

1 tsp cumin

½ tsp garlic powder

½ tsp salt, plus more to taste

½ tsp black pepper, plus more to taste

1 lb (454 g) chicken thighs

1 (4-oz [113-g]) can diced green chiles

1 cup (240 ml) salsa verde

4 cups (960 ml) chicken broth

1 cup (240 ml) unsweetened coconut or almond milk

½ cup (73 g) raw cashews

Avocado, lime wedges and chopped cilantro, for garnish

In a large pot over medium-high heat, heat the avocado oil. Add the onion, bell pepper and carrots and sauté for about 5 minutes, or until the vegetables are tender-crisp. Add the cumin, garlic powder, salt and pepper to the pot and stir. Add the chicken thighs. Pour in the diced green chiles, salsa verde and chicken broth and stir to combine. Bring the soup to a low boil and cover. Cook for 15 minutes, or until the chicken is cooked through, stirring occasionally.

In a blender, combine the coconut milk and cashews and blend until super smooth, about 1 to 2 minutes.

Reduce the heat to low and bring the soup to a simmer. Remove the chicken from the pot and chop into bite-sized pieces. Stir the chopped chicken and cashew cream into the soup.

Season with additional salt and pepper to taste. Serve hot, garnished with avocado, lime wedges and chopped cilantro.

INSALATA DI ANITPASTI

Let's take an antipasto platter and make it a salad! This is a no-cook dish in which Italian appetizer favorites come together to make a full meal. With savory meats, fresh vegetables, fatty olives and the perfectly tangy Italian herb dressing, you'll forget all about the main course. This quick salad is a favorite for nights when we want to "fridge forage" and can't be bothered to heat up the kitchen.

YIELD: 4 SERVINGS
PREP TIME: 10 MINUTES
COOKING TIME: 0 MINUTES

FOR THE DRESSING

3 tbsp (45 ml) olive oil

1 tbsp (15 ml) balsamic vinegar

1 tbsp (15 ml) red wine vinegar

1 tsp Dijon mustard

1 tsp minced garlic

½ tsp salt

½ tsp black pepper

½ tsp dried Italian herb seasoning

FOR THE SALAD

6 cups (450 g) romaine lettuce, chopped

½ cup (90 g) mixed Greek olives, pitted

1 cup (149 g) grape tomatoes, halved

1 (6-oz [170-g]) jar roasted red peppers, drained and sliced

1 (6-oz [170-g]) jar artichoke hearts, drained and chopped

4 oz (113 g) thick-cut salami, chopped

4 oz (113 g) prosciutto

¼ cup (15 g) fresh chopped parsley

To make the dressing: In a small bowl, whisk together the olive oil, balsamic, red wine vinegar, Dijon, garlic, salt, pepper and Italian herb seasoning. Transfer to the refrigerator until ready to serve.

To make the salad: Arrange the salads by dividing the ingredients equally among four bowls. Top with the Italian dressing to taste (I like about 2 tablespoons [30 ml] on each salad) and serve chilled.

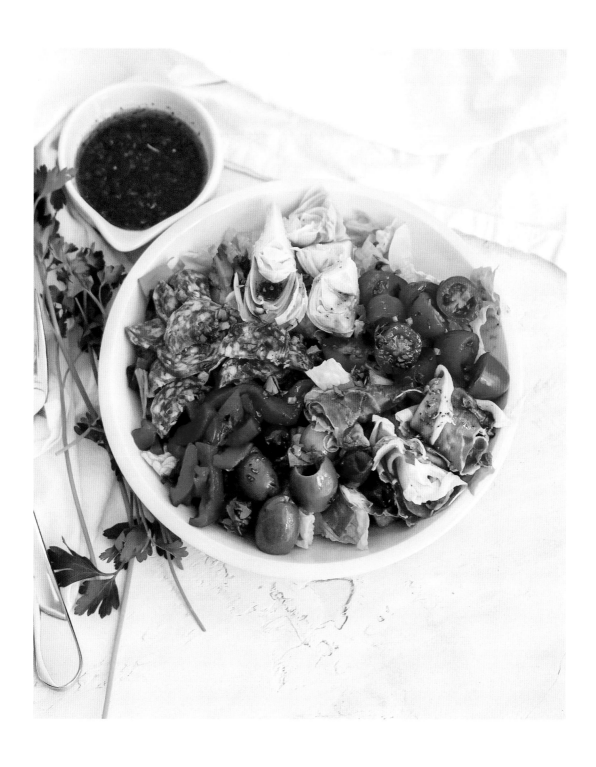

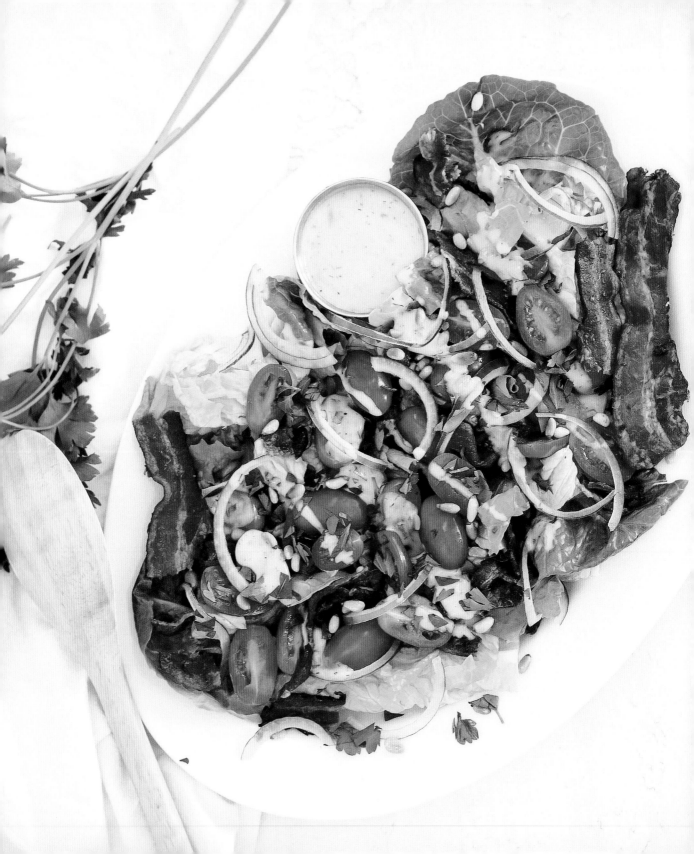

BLT SALAD WITH CRISPY OVEN BACON

Oven bacon is a longtime staple for me, and the trick to getting it perfectly crispy every time, with no splatter or mess: a cold oven! Cook yours up and serve it "BLT" style in this fresh salad loaded up with all of the toppings for perfect texture and flavor in every bite.

YIELD: 4 SERVINGS
PREP TIME: 5 MINUTES
COOKING TIME: 25 MINUTES

12 oz (340 g) bacon

16 romaine heart leaves

½ cup (68 g) pine nuts

½ small red onion, thinly sliced

2 cups (298 g) grape or cherry tomatoes, halved

¼ cup (15 g) fresh parsley, finely chopped

Paleo-friendly ranch dressing

Line a baking sheet with parchment paper. Arrange the bacon slices in a single layer and transfer to a cold oven. Once the bacon is in, set the oven to heat to 425°F (218°C), and set a timer for 20 minutes. Cook up to 5 minutes more to ensure the bacon is crispy. Once cooked, transfer the bacon slices to a cooling rack lined with paper towels until ready to serve.

To serve, arrange the romaine heart leaves on the bottom of a large serving platter. Top with the cooked bacon (crumbled or whole), pine nuts, red onion, tomatoes, chopped parsley and ranch dressing.

QUICK TIP: You can make your own Paleo ranch dressing, or go ahead and grab one in-store or online! There are so many great options now, many even shelf-stable, for keeping on hand in the pantry.

SPICY-SWEET THAI BEEF SALAD WITH TOASTED COCONUT CASHEWS

This salad was inspired by a favorite of ours from a restaurant we used to go to all of the time for the best fresh salads made to order. It starts with a Thai-inspired dressing-marinade hybrid. It's what you'll use to flavor up the grilled steak and also what brings the whole thing together at the end. My favorite part? The spicy-sweet toasted coconut cashews! They add the perfect crunch.

YIELD: 4 SERVINGS
PREP TIME: 10 MINUTES
COOKING TIME: 20 MINUTES

1 lb (454 g) sirloin steak

3 tbsp (45 ml) lime juice

3 tbsp (45 ml) coconut aminos

3 tbsp (45 ml) avocado oil

1 tsp minced garlic

1 tsp minced ginger

1 tsp red curry paste

½ cup (65 g) raw cashew pieces

⅓ cup (31 g) unsweetened shredded coconut

2 tsp (10 ml) honey

¼ tsp red pepper flakes

8 loosely packed cups (363 g) spring mix

½ medium red bell pepper, thinly sliced, for garnish

¼ cup (12 g) thinly sliced scallion, for garnish

¼ cup (4 g) cilantro, roughly chopped, for garnish

½ cup (20 g) basil leaves, sliced thin, for garnish

Pat the steak dry with a paper towel and set aside. In a large shallow bowl or glass dish, whisk the lime juice, coconut aminos, avocado oil, garlic, ginger and red curry paste. Transfer half of the mixture to a small bowl to use as your dressing. Add the steak to the large bowl with the remaining marinade until ready to cook.

Heat a grill pan or cast-iron skillet over medium-high heat. Put the marinated steak in the hot pan and grill for 5 minutes per side. Transfer to a cutting board and allow the steak to rest for 10 minutes. Slice thin against the grain.

While the steak cooks, heat a small pan over medium-low. Put in the cashews, coconut, honey and red pepper flakes. Cook, stirring occasionally, for 7 to 8 minutes, or until toasted and golden brown.

To serve, arrange the spring mix in bowls or on a large serving plate. Top with the steak and toasted coconut cashews. Pour the dressing over top, and garnish with red bell pepper, scallion, cilantro and basil.

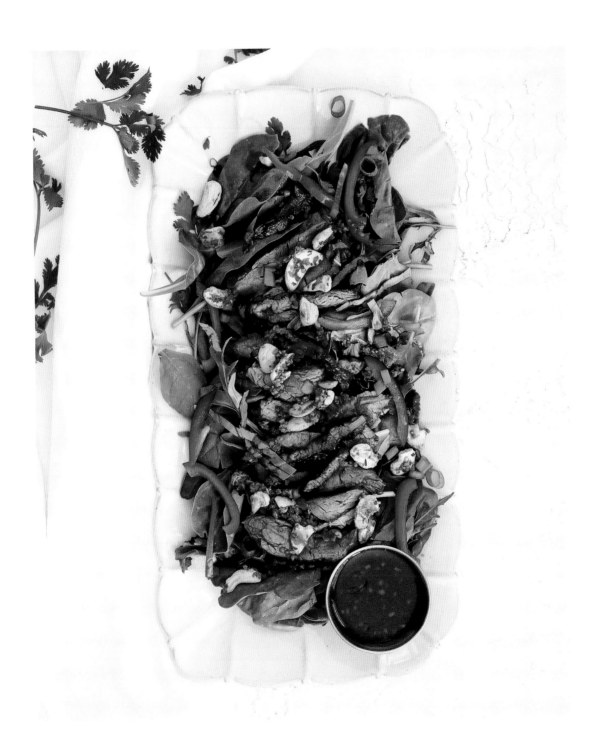

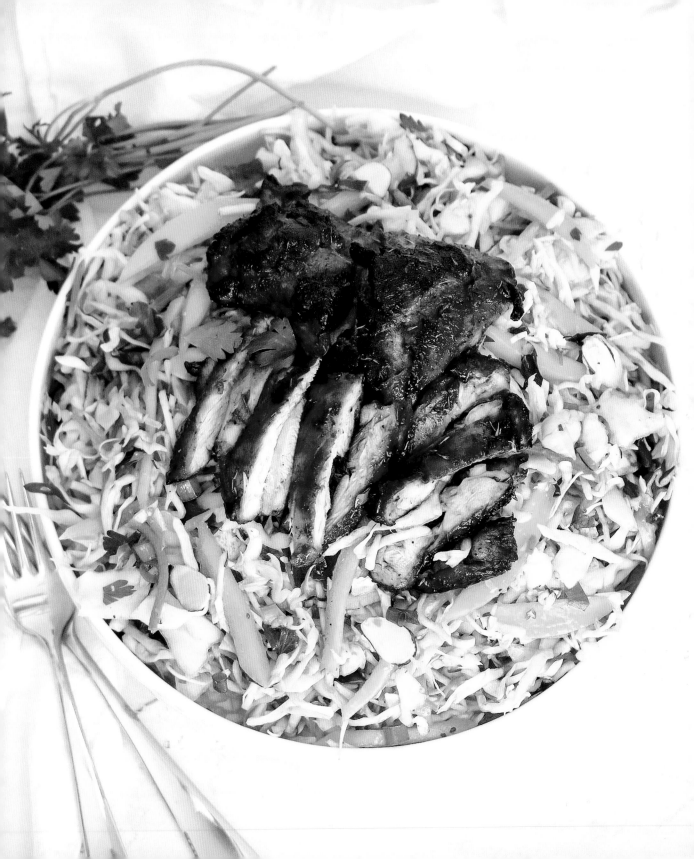

JAMAICAN JERK CHICKEN THIGHS WITH TROPICAL SLAW

I love it when a dish truly transports my taste buds to another time and place—and that is exactly what this one does. One bite, and you'll be sitting on a tropical beach with the tastes of Jamaica. The marinade on these caramelized chicken thighs is thick, sticky, savory, sweet and rich with warm flavors—it's truly like no other. Serve them up over the light citrusy slaw with fresh mango, jalapeño and scallion and feel the island vibes!

YIELD: 4 SERVINGS
PREP TIME: 10 MINUTES
COOKING TIME: 12 MINUTES

FOR THE CHICKEN

2 tbsp (30 ml) coconut aminos

2 tbsp (30 ml) honey

2 tbsp (30 ml) olive oil

2 tsp (4 g) onion powder

½ tsp garlic powder

1 tsp cinnamon

1 tsp dried thyme

½ tsp salt

½ tsp black pepper

¼ tsp cayenne pepper (optional, if you like some heat)

¼ tsp nutmeg

¼ tsp cloves

1 lb (454 g) boneless, skinless chicken thighs

FOR THE SLAW

2 tbsp (30 ml) honey

2 tbsp (30 ml) lemon juice

2 tbsp (30 ml) olive oil

1 tbsp (15 ml) Dijon mustard

1 tsp minced garlic

1 tsp hot sauce

6 cups (1.2 kg) coleslaw mix

1 large mango, peeled and julienned

½ cup (72 g) roasted sliced almonds

¼ cup (12 g) thinly sliced scallion

¼ cup (15 g) chopped parsley

½ jalapeño, minced

½ tsp salt

To make the chicken: In a large shallow bowl or baking dish, combine the coconut aminos, honey, olive oil, onion powder, garlic powder, cinnamon, thyme, salt, pepper, cayenne (if using), nutmeg and cloves. Whisk until smooth, then add the chicken thighs to the marinade. Let it sit for 5 minutes while you prep the slaw.

To make the slaw: In a bowl large enough to fit the slaw, combine the honey, lemon juice, olive oil, Dijon, garlic and hot sauce. Whisk until smooth. Add the coleslaw mix, mango, almonds, scallion, parsley, jalapeño and salt. Toss to evenly coat the slaw with the dressing. I like to use a large bowl with a fitted lid, then shake to toss quickly. Refrigerate until ready to serve.

Heat a grill pan or large skillet over medium-high heat. Add the chicken thighs to the hot pan, and cook for 5 minutes, or until browned. Flip, and cook for 5 to 7 minutes more, or until the internal temperature of the thickest part of the chicken reads 165°F (74°C).

Serve the hot chicken thighs over the tropical slaw.

GREEK CHICKEN SALAD WITH LEMON-HERB VINAIGRETTE

If you're looking for crowd-pleasing flavors with a beautiful presentation, you have come to the right place. This bright Greek salad is bursting with fresh lemon and balanced out perfectly by the savory herb-roasted chicken. Think Greek gyro meat, but cooked quickly in the oven in its own marinade to really amp up the flavor and juiciness. Try this served family style, or prep for lunches in small containers!

YIELD: 4 SERVINGS
PREP TIME: 10 MINUTES
COOKING TIME: 20 MINUTES

FOR THE CHICKEN

½ lb (227 g) boneless, skinless chicken breasts or tenders
1 tbsp (15 ml) olive oil
1½ tsp (7 ml) red wine vinegar
1 clove garlic, minced
1 tsp dried oregano
½ tsp salt
¼ tsp black pepper
¼ tsp paprika
¼ tsp garlic powder
¼ tsp onion powder

FOR THE DRESSING

¼ cup (60 ml) olive oil
Zest of 1 lemon
Juice of 1 lemon
2 tsp (10 ml) Dijon mustard
2 cloves garlic, minced
1 tsp dried Italian herb seasoning
½ tsp honey
½ tsp salt
¼ tsp black pepper

FOR THE SALAD

4 packed cups mixed greens
1 small cucumber, sliced
½ cup (75 g) halved grape tomatoes
½ small red onion, thinly sliced
½ cup (90 g) mixed Greek olives, pitted
½ cup (120 ml) zucchini hummus (optional, see page 96)

To make the chicken: Preheat the oven to 425°F (218°C). Line a baking sheet with parchment paper and set aside. If using whole chicken breasts, slice them in half so they will cook faster. Pat dry with a paper towel. In a medium mixing bowl, combine the olive oil, red wine vinegar, minced garlic, oregano, salt, pepper, paprika, garlic powder and onion powder. Add the chicken and toss to coat. Let the chicken sit for 5 minutes before transferring to the lined baking sheet. Transfer to the oven and bake for 15 to 20 minutes, or until an internal temperature reads 165°F (74°C).

To make the dressing: While the chicken bakes, in a medium bowl, whisk together the olive oil, lemon zest, lemon juice, Dijon, garlic, Italian herb seasoning, honey, salt and pepper until smooth and combined. You can also put the ingredients in a Mason jar with a tight-fitting lid and shake well until emulsified to speed up the process.

To assemble the salad: Arrange the mixed greens in four bowls or on a large serving platter. Top with sliced cucumber, halved tomatoes, sliced red onion, olives and a scoop of hummus (if using). Slice the cooked chicken and layer over top. Drizzle with the lemon-herb vinaigrette and enjoy.

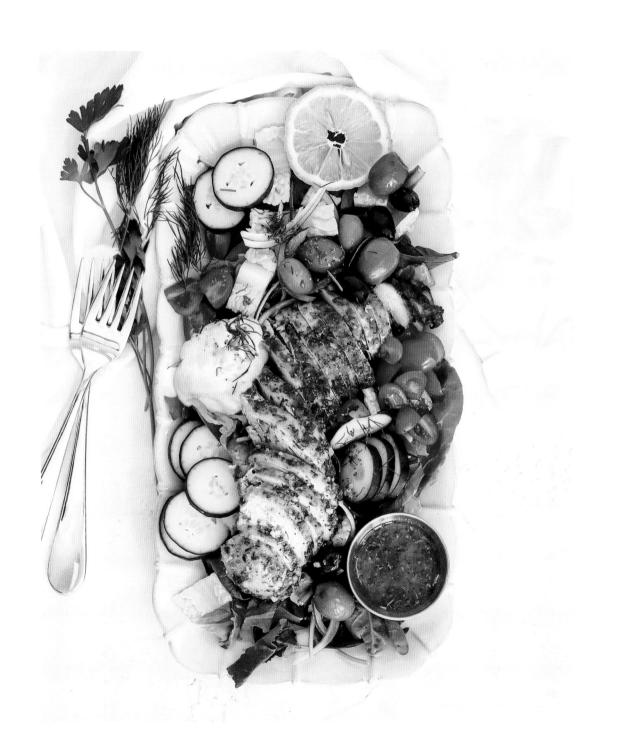

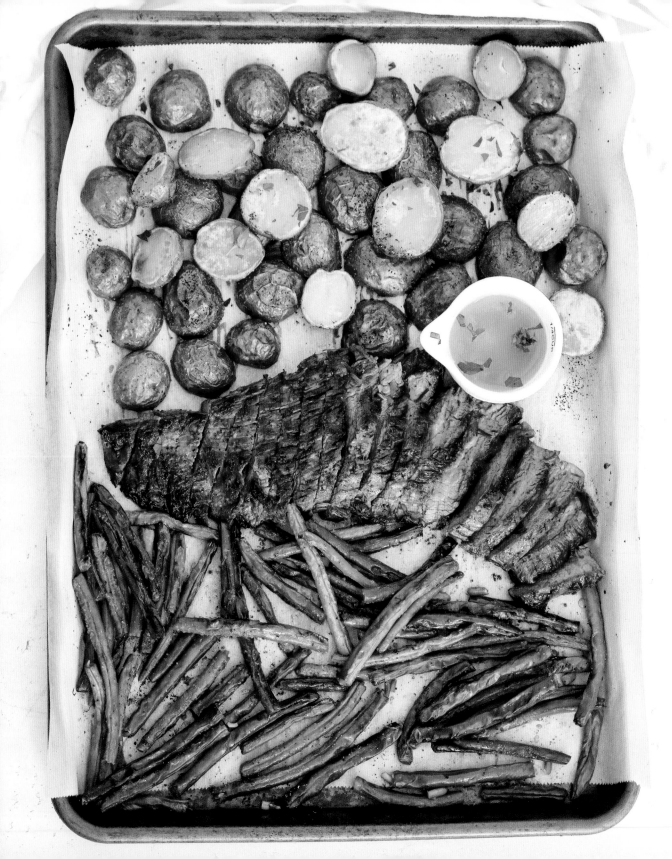

ACKNOWLEDGMENTS

To my husband, Dathan, for being the best partner and teammate a girl could ask for. Thank you for pushing me when I doubt myself, saying "yes" to all of my wild ideas and always putting our family first. None of this would be a reality without your physical and emotional support and your epic taste-testing abilities. I love you so much!

To my parents, Larry and Julie: Kobe Bryant once said, "My parents are my backbone. Still are. They're the only group that will support you if you score zero or you score 40." I couldn't agree more. Thank you for being my biggest cheerleaders, no matter what. Your support means everything!

To the team at Page Street Publishing, for your meticulous work, warm interactions and endless patience with this overwhelmed mom of two under two. It's been an absolute pleasure completing yet another beautiful book with you. Sixty brand new recipes each done in 30 minutes or less sounded nearly impossible, but I knew I couldn't say no to the challenge. Thank you for having such faith in me! These are the recipes I needed in my own life!

Finally, to my community of Just Jessie B readers and friends: Here we are again—cookbook number two! This truly wouldn't have happened without your love and enthusiasm for *The Simple Paleo Kitchen*. You all continue to blow me away with your constant support, and I'm eternally grateful. I cannot wait to see you whipping up these recipes in your kitchens in no time flat!

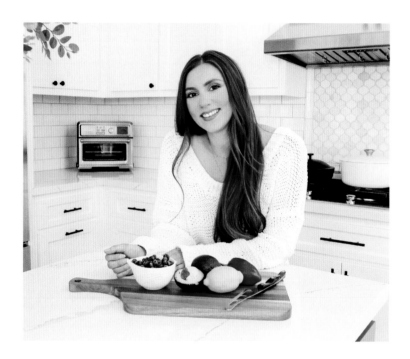

ABOUT THE AUTHOR

Jessie Bittner is the author of *The Simple Paleo Kitchen* as well as the creator, blogger and photographer behind Just Jessie B, a food and lifestyle blog full of simple, mostly Paleo recipes and inspiration for living a clean and healthy life. She specializes in simple, comfort food–style, gluten- and dairy-free creations that the whole family will love—little ones and non-Paleo folks included.

Jessie's love for Paleo eating and cooking began in grad school, where she earned her master's degree in speech language pathology. She has spent several years following her other passion: working with children with special needs, including speech and language disorders.

Jessie now puts her love of food and helping children to work at home, running her own business and raising her sons. Jessie lives in Morgan Hill, California, with her husband, Dathan, and their two boys, Hudson and Ford.

INDEX